Turning Lead Into Gold

Turning Lead Into Gold

How Heavy Metal Poisoning Can Affect
Your Child, And How To Prevent
And Treat It

Nancy Hallaway, RN
and Zigurts Strauts, MD

New Star Books
Vancouver
1995

Published by New Star Books Ltd., 2504 York Avenue, Vancouver, B.C., Canada V6K 1E3. All rights reserved. No part of this work may be reproduced or used in any form or by any means — graphic, electronic, or mechanical — without the prior written permission of the publisher. Any request for photocopying or other reprographic copying must be sent in writing to the Canadian Copyright Licensing Agency (CANCOPY), 6 Adelaide Street East, Suite 900, Toronto, ON M5C 1H6.

Publication of this book is made possible by grants from the Canada Council and the Cultural Services Branch, Province of British Columbia.

Printed and bound in Canada by Best Book Manufacturers
Cover design by Tom Moore
1 2 3 4 5   99 98 97 96 95

Canadian Cataloguing in Publication Data
Hallaway, Nancy, 1959-
  Turning lead into gold

  ISBN 0-921586-51-5
  1. Heavy metals — Toxicology.   2. Heavy metals — Environmental aspects. 3. Pediatric toxicology   I. Strauts, Zigurts, 1947-   II. Title.
RA1231.M52H34 1995   363.17′9   C95-910559-X

My heartfelt thanks and gratitude to Judi Langley.
You were my first shining star! You helped me to believe there was
a light at the end of the tunnel.
Also to Elizabeth Forrest, Kim Pattison, and Steve Cunningham
for giving me the opportunity to find the light.
Most of all to Zigurts Strauts
for having the courage and insight to challenge and persevere.
You are responsible for changing our family's entire future.
You provided our miracle.
N.H.

To all the wonderful mothers and fathers
who forever give to their children unconditional love.
They are our hope.
Z.S.

Contents

Prologue

In November 1992 I began to write my story of life with attention deficit, hyperactive children with autistic tendencies. Writing my story was to be the start of the healing process, the process of accepting my children's and family's unfortunate fate. Somehow, putting the words on paper helped resolve some of the anger and the pain I was feeling. It let me acknowledge the problem. It also made me realize that I had to get on with life despite my children's problems. I had to make the best of it.

In 1993 I became a patient of Dr. Zigurts Strauts. Even though I was seeing him for my own health problems, he quite unexpectedly recognized the underlying cause of my children's problems. Together we identified a major childhood epidemic of metal poisoning and, after testing and treating many children from our community and others for toxic metals, we are observing some remarkable changes in their condition and behavior upon detoxification.

We naively proceeded to bring our discoveries to the attention of the appropriate authorities in government and the medical profession, hoping to get the word out to other parents, but were met with only shock, denial, resistance, and disbelief.

For these reasons, we decided to write the story and share our experiences directly with those who need this information. This has been an extremely hard manuscript to write. It required both of us to sacrifice our families' privacy and confidentiality. We had to expose a vulnerable side of our own dysfunctional personal lives.

But we could not withhold this critical medical information that could improve the lives of hundreds of thousands, perhaps millions of young children and their families. We felt that, ethically, not telling our story could be the equivalent of child neglect and medical irresponsibility.

Zigurts and I have both put our personal lives on hold to get this information out. We feel that we must provide families with what might be the missing key to their children's developmental problems, the missing key that might provide some understanding, relief, and recovery.

Much of this story is told by me, but the work in the manuscript was a dual effort on the part of myself and Zigurts, along with a strong third presence — our editor, Audrey McClellan. This is a book that could only be possible with both my personal story and Zigurts' medical expertise, amalgamated into one by Audrey's excellent advice and editing skills.

Nancy Hallaway
May 22, 1995

1

Just One More Month . . .

"It's a boy, Mrs. Hallaway," exclaimed the doctor. "And there's another one coming right now. Look at that. Two perfect baby boys. Aren't you going to be busy."

Little did he know I was going to be much more than just busy. Cameron and Brett were indeed two perfect-looking, healthy little baby boys. They were born three weeks early on March 22, 1988, delivered by caesarean section, weighing seven pounds, four ounces and six pounds, ten ounces — almost fifteen pounds of babies!

The twins were a real treat for the first six weeks. They nursed — they slept. We were proud of how well we were coping with the twins and our fifteen-month-old daughter, all in cribs and diapers. The boys were so passive and easy that we were able to focus almost all of our attention on helping our daughter adjust to the new arrivals. Life was wonderful.

Then, after week six, the "twins from hell" woke up. They nursed every three to four hours. They stayed awake almost all of the time. And they needed constant attention. In the night, one twin would wake up the other, and then their sister would join us. I was up all night with my wonderful family. I must admit, I enjoyed it. Although I could have used some extra sleep, I was proud of my children and I loved to be with them.

As the first year whipped by, I found myself getting a little more rest as the twins established a regular pattern of napping, sleeping, and feeding. When times were tough and I felt like I was running out of steam, I would talk myself into believing that things would be better if we could get past one more month . . . just one more month!

During their first year the twins were extremely healthy. They didn't have any problems with illness or colds. They were growing like weeds and getting chubby. They were happy, nursed well, moved around like crazy, and were so cute. Everything seemed normal though, in retrospect, there were some signs that the twins were having difficulties during that first year. It became apparent they had a severe separation anxiety. Several times I called in a babysitter and tried to get out for awhile, but the job was too difficult for the sitter. The boys would cry from the time I left until I returned home. I couldn't leave them, unless they were already asleep, without mayhem breaking out. Soon it became impossible to get out at all. Oh, well . . . just one more month, I thought.

The boys' motor skills appeared to be developing normally. They sat alone at five months old. They crawled by seven or eight months. By ten months they were trying to walk, holding onto furniture or the odd spare hand. They were interested in toys and would watch cars driving by. They appeared to recognize all of our immediate family members. They smiled, they laughed, they played and teased. Speech was not coming as quickly or as easily as it had for our daughter. Actually, speech was not coming at all. They say that twins are often in their own world, that they have an unspoken language or make up their own language. These guys sure did seem to understand each other. We suspected that this was the reason for their language delay.

By the time the twins were eighteen months old the separation anxiety, which we had expected would disappear, was getting worse. The twins were upset and anxious about almost everything. Their pattern of napping, sleeping, and eating, which had taken so long to get established, was falling apart. They were awake almost all of the time, and from the first minute of waking they were crying and upset the whole day. It was hard work trying to keep them happy. A drive in the car was about the only thing that soothed and relaxed them, and I would often bundle them up and take them for a ride around the neighborhood. Over the next six months their appetites diminished and they began to have frequent, loose, bowel movements. We passed these symptoms off as teething problems. Our days were filled with unorganized chaos, but any parent with three children in bottles, diapers, and cribs would probably tell you that.

Cam and Brett were also beginning to exhibit unusual fears of new things and experiences. If we went into a store, an elevator, an office, or a car wash, they became frightened and upset, getting so worked up that they were completely out of control . . . screaming, thrashing, crying, and biting themselves. These little twins were distressed by anything that they weren't familiar with, but because we were so housebound, they weren't familiar with much of anything. We thought perhaps it was just another unusual stage in "twinness."

They couldn't stand anyone new coming to our house, even family members. They would take my hand and try to drag me away from company. Anybody else entering our house triggered bedlam.

By this time the twins were also ripping their clothes off and having grotesque episodes of fecal smearing. They would cover their cribs with feces, fling it up on the walls, smear it through their hair, all over their bodies, and cover their toys with it. It was so bad that most of the time I could only look at the mess and wonder where in the heck to begin cleaning. The worst part was, this was not a rare occurrence. It was happening almost daily. I wondered for a while if it was being used as a tool to keep visitors away. It sure worked.

As the smearing catastrophes continued, I started to dress the twins in clothing like jumpsuits that I could put on backwards in hopes that they wouldn't be able to get them off. I soon had to resort to pinning their clothes shut at the back. Before long, even that didn't work. The twins pulled all of their clothing off, or tore it apart if they had to. There was no way of keeping them dressed and nothing that we could do to prevent the grotesque "accidents" except to monitor them constantly.

We also had to start thinking about what might happen when the twins were able to get outside by themselves. Our house was on Mountain Highway, a busy road in North Vancouver, British Columbia, near a main intersection in the Lynn Valley area. There was way too much traffic — crossing the street could be extremely difficult — an excess of noise and car exhaust fumes, and too many sirens. We envisioned huge problems once the twins could unlock the front door. It was not safe there, so we decided to build our dream home in a quiet subdivision a few miles away.

The twins were almost two years old when we moved into our new house. We still thought they would grow out of their problems, though we realized they were quite delayed developmentally. Certainly they were incredibly hyperactive, hyperanxious, and a hyper-pain-in-the-ass! They scattered everything that they touched and there seemed to be no way for us to discipline them. We weren't sure they understood anything that we said, and couldn't tell if they knew their own names. They certainly didn't respond to our verbal attempts to discipline them, and we knew that hitting them wouldn't work. These little guys had no fear of punishment. They didn't seem to feel pain. A spank made no difference to them. They had no common sense, were extremely impulsive, and had no self control. Nothing appeared to make any sense to them.

They still had no appetite, and would only drink fluids. They didn't appreciate the typical things that little kids like (crackers, cookies, fruit), and were getting skinny. Our family doctor thought it could still be teething. Probably just a stage. And the language delay? "Don't worry about the language delay. Why, my nephew didn't talk until he was five years old and he's a lawyer now!" the doctor said. So we tried not to worry. We just persevered.

The next couple of years were, without a doubt, the worst of our lives. It was difficult just getting through a day with the twins, and since they were terrible sleepers, the day often went on until one or two in the morning. They would tear the house to pieces, scream, smear feces, shred books, scatter toys, and fling food all around the house. It was impossible to keep the house clean, impossible to teach the twins any kind of typical house etiquette. They could not comprehend the simplest instructions. They were excessively hyperactive and they literally bounced off the walls. Not only that, they ate the walls. They actually bit holes into the drywall. They unlocked the doors and jumped out of windows. Once on the street, the twins grabbed at the tires of moving vehicles. They would take (and destroy) neighbors' possessions that were left outside. They would scale the seven-foot back fence, jump down the other side, and escape through the neighboring cul de sac . . . naked! They never looked back, they never thought about dangers or how they would return home. They required 24-hour supervision to protect them from themselves.

At night the twins would escape from their cribs (they would not stay in a bed, let alone sleep in one). Of course this meant we didn't get any sleep either. We resorted to dropping the crib mattresses to the floor, building a one-foot base around the bottom of their cribs and another one-foot frame around the top. It didn't take long for them to figure out how to shake the crib back and forth hard enough to tip the entire frame over and escape. They could get out of the house before we knew they were awake. We were desperate, so after careful consideration, my husband and I decided that we would have to lock them in their rooms at night for their own protection. We also had to lock shut their windows so that they wouldn't jump out of them. It seemed like an awful thing to do but we really cared for these demented little kids and were always concerned about their safety.

Day by day I struggled on, looking after the house and kids, and working the odd night shift as a registered nurse at the local hospital. This was a problem, though, as the twins would run away while I tried to sleep after my night shifts. I would have to get up and search for them, and let me tell you, to lose a child who has run away naked and doesn't know his name is terrifying.

My husband hated the way we had to live. I guess I did too. We always thought that the twins would snap out of it. But that wasn't happening. In fact, it was getting much worse. The twins were constantly screaming, crying, throwing items, and destroying our furniture. They broke almost everything we owned. "No" meant nothing to them and, as I mentioned, punishment of any form accomplished nothing. I remember vividly one relative telling us, "You just have to start hitting them." Hit them? We knew that we could have broken every bone in their little bodies and it still would not have registered with these kids. There were several other people who told us, "All kids are the same, you have to discipline these little guys more." It was obvious that we were seen as inadequate parents. We knew that we weren't, but we didn't have any explanation as to why these kids were so damn difficult to deal with. We tried harder than any other parent that I was aware of and never got anywhere with them. It was obvious to both my husband and myself that the twins didn't have any power over their hyperactivity, impulsiveness, their need to climb, run, jump, destroy things, and escape. Something appeared to be playing a cruel joke on their central nervous system and their overall mental functions.

We hung on and kept repairing the damage that these destructive little guys caused. Soon there was very little left in our house to repair. The twins spent hours tearing everything apart. They jabbed knives and screwdrivers into the walls. They smashed eggs and dishes. They would not sit at the table for meals; they hardly ever wanted meals. And at three years old they hadn't even attempted spoonfeeding themselves yet. They finally did begin to eat some solid foods again — nachos with cheese, chicken, and bacon. What a diet, eh? But they wouldn't eat any other food. It didn't matter what or how you presented it, and you couldn't get anywhere by trying to force them to eat. So I was resigned to feeding them lots of whatever it was that they would eat at the current time. Most of the time they preferred fluids to a solid diet, but only apple juice or milk. They wouldn't touch anything else, not even water — unless it was out of the toilet.

That brings me to another point: they had this big thing for toilets — just so long as they didn't have to go to the bathroom in them. It terrified them to sit on one. They refused to use the toilet except to splash in it, climb in it, even drink from it if they could. It was completely disgusting, not to mention a huge inconvenience.

You can guess by now that my husband and I were getting burned out. These miserable little boys gave us no space. Because of their separation anxiety, we could seldom use babysitters. They still cried for hours when I stepped out the door. I felt terrible hearing them wailing while I left and knowing I would have to contend with the mess and confusion when I returned home. It was not worth going out. They still tore every bit of their clothing off as fast as I could put it on. They hated to be confined in clothes. They ran around naked almost all of the time, despite my buying them every type of clothing that I thought they might like. They continued to have bowel movements wherever they happened to be at the time and they continued to jump in the excrement, smear it and fling it on the walls, into the furniture, into their hair.

I remember having my sister and her husband over for

lunch in our new house. One of the twins stood right beside my newly acquired brother-in-law, defecated on the floor beside him while he was eating his lunch, then jumped into it and ran through the house. What can you say? Whoops!? We had four toilets, for God's sake!

There was nothing rewarding about this period of time except sleep. And that was a scarce commodity. Boy, how I wished this would end.

2

The Worst Years:
Struggling for Control

Ever had a child that tried to jump out of a car travelling across a bridge at 90 kilometres per hour with traffic moving just as fast on both sides of you? Or one that ran out to touch a moving train as it went by? How about one that tried to jump into the killer whale tank at the aquarium? One who stripped off all his clothes in front of company and got an erection playing with his aunt's toes? I had *two* kids like this!

It was obvious by the twins' third birthday that they were not getting better — they appeared to be worse. Every day was one big hectic blur. Anxiety was high in the Hallaway household; our patience was wearing thin and so were our tempers. By this time we had alienated most of our friends and some of our family. We couldn't handle any extra stress.

The boys turned three on March 22, 1991. They still had never had a real birthday party. They had no friends. We had no company except for a couple of relatives who could stand visiting us for a short duration. If chaos happened, we all just laughed it off.

By this time I realized how dysfunctional and abnormal our situation was, and I couldn't stand it anymore. I was tired of doing all of the housework and looking after the kids. Nothing ever got finished, so my husband and I decided to hire a nanny. Maybe this would give us a much-needed break and let us start to live again. I contacted a nanny service and within one month we had a wonderful nanny. Claire started working with us on my birthday, April 4, 1991.

Claire was deeply religious, very quiet, and a sincere woman with a heart of gold. She was kind, gentle, and extremely patient — exactly what we needed, as our kids sure required special considerations. Delegating some of the responsibility for their care was a slow process. The boys didn't take kindly to a new caregiver, even someone who lived with us. For the first while it seemed best to make as few waves as possible. I would only leave the house when they were safely asleep. Otherwise it was pandemonium. But the ability to finally get out was such a treat for me, it didn't matter when I had to do it.

I don't know how we pulled it off, but Claire and I managed to make it through the long, hot summer of 1991. Despite the fact that there were now two of us to look after the three children, they were still too much work. My husband was content to escape to his job as a paramedic as often as he could, so Claire and I struggled together to keep the kids alive and growing. It was a difficult and ungratifying job. We tried to take the kids places but it was clear every place we went that the boys were not socially appropriate. Their bizarre behavior and odd mannerisms made them stick out like sore thumbs in public. They continued to strip out of their clothing in spite of all our efforts to keep the stuff on. We ended up leaving almost every place we went with unhappy, combative, and uncooperative children, and with Claire and me completely pissed off. Everything was just too hard. It was easier to stay home and stay isolated.

Life was becoming unbearably painful. Our family life was the pits, our marriage was showing signs of strain, and it was obvious that our daughter (who was only fifteen months older than the twins) was becoming emotionally crippled. We all had difficulty coping with the twins, but our daughter's self-esteem was particularly deflated by their socially inappropriate actions and behavior. She showed signs of increasing insecurity and was afraid to go to bed at night. Her one special wish was that her brothers would be "normal" one day and could talk and play with her.

When the twins were almost three and a half we finally consulted a pediatrician to see if they might be having more than the usual twin problems. We had our first appointment with the new doctor on August 22, 1991. During that visit he stated that he had seen only one child worse than ours in his 25 years as a pediatrician. It was blunt, but kind of funny, and we were relieved to hear it. Now we knew that it wasn't poor parenting skills. The doctor stated that the twins were clearly impossible and would need some investigating. For the time being, though, as they were truly hyperactive and also had an obvious attention deficit disorder, he recommended that we try a medication called Ritalin to improve their concentration and, therefore, their attention span.

My husband and I were relieved but shocked. It was nice to have something definite that we could try. On the other hand . . . Ritalin? It was so controversial. It was not recommended for children under ten years old. But we were desperate.

I figured if we were going to try something as drastic as Ritalin on our three-year-old twins, I had darn well better be around to oversee it. I took a leave of absence from work and stepped down from my nursing career indefinitely, planning to dedicate as much time as necessary to sorting out my children's problems.

On August 24, 1991, we started the twins on Ritalin, despite warnings from my husband's medical colleagues and our pharmacist. It was a difficult decision to make and abide by. When we picked up the prescription for Ritalin, the pharmacist told us that the drug was not recommended for young children. She called the doctor's office to check that he hadn't made a mistake.

It was extremely hard to get them to take the medication,

but it was worth it. Ritalin is a bitter-tasting pill, so we had to crush it and hide it in their milk or juice. Sometimes they would taste it and send the cup of fluid flying across the room. Other times they would drink it down and within half an hour would be semi-manageable. Unfortunately, these boys wouldn't eat jam, honey, or other things that you could hide pills in, so there was little choice but to hide it in their drinks.

Giving Cam and Brett this drug was an eye opener. Within a few days we discovered, for the first time, that these kids did know their names. And their attention spans improved a small, but significant, amount. Even with the new medication, the twins remained uptight and anxious, perhaps more than before. Loud noises terrified them and made them extremely agitated. Simple things like a dog barking or a car engine starting would frighten them badly. But they finally looked at us when we called their respective names (though they didn't understand anything else that we were saying). We felt that even this was some progress.

Our pediatrician also arranged for us to have the twins assessed at Vancouver's Sunny Hill Health Centre for Children, which specializes in diagnosing children with disabilities. This was to be a definitive assessment, or so we thought. Unfortunately the boys were so uncooperative that the examination could only be done visually, and what should have been two days of tests was reduced to two hours of incomplete, unsuccessful examinations. The twins didn't pay any attention to the doctor, a pediatrician specializing in children's behavioral and mental development.

The doctor stated that they did indeed have severe attention problems and were extremely hyperactive and agitated. He also commented on their limited and unusual eye contact — they made no eye contact with any of the diagnostic team (this included the pediatrician, a speech pathologist, and a psychologist) and they seldom made eye contact with us. He mentioned that they had very complex behavior problems (I remember thinking, when he said this, "No shit, Sherlock! Why do you think we're here?"). His diagnosis: attention deficit disorder with severe hyperactivity and probable autism. And his advice was, "Continue with the prescribed Ritalin if you think it is helping. We will reassess them at another time when their behavior is more controlled." He also commended us for hanging in there with them.

I couldn't believe it. For some reason I had thought that this place was going to give us some answers on how to care for and cope with these children. Instead they put us through two hours of hell trying to look after our demented little children while they unsuccessfully tested them. Then the doctor reiterated what we already knew, added a new label — probable autism — and suggested that we continue doing what we were already doing until they were better controlled. How were they going to get better controlled? These children were beyond control. Even with the prescribed medication, this was the best behavior we could get out of these kids. We were no farther ahead. We had no direction. We were getting plain pissed off. This was definitely not much fun. And now we had another label attached to their diagnosis.

When the boys' pediatrician realized how upset we were over this failed appointment, he set us up with a child psychiatrist at the British Columbia's Children's Hospital, an acute care hospital for children in Vancouver. This proved to be a step in the right direction. The psychiatrist suggested another diagnosis for our twins, pervasive developmental disorder. He also recognized that Ritalin was making the twins more anxious. He prescribed Anafranil, a tricyclic anti-depressant used widely in the United States for attentional problems, to be given in place of Ritalin. Without too much hesitation, we started the boys on Anafranil. It definitely had a better effect than Ritalin. They started to sleep again at night, and went to bed at a reasonable time — for about one month. Unfortunately, after the month had passed they seemed to be conditioned to the medication and had insomnia once again.

Despite the medication, every single day with Cam and Brett was still frustrating. It was hard enough putting up with the boys' mischief; anything extra that occurred in a day pushed Claire and me into overload. I was run down and always tired. Claire's shift ended at 4:30 p.m. so she could close her door to our lunacy. For me, the shift continued into the night. The twins' sleeping habits had become poor again, and our daughter's were also deteriorating. Each child was up several times a night, crying and unable to fall back to sleep for hours. Our daughter was anxious and upset a lot of the time, as were we all. She would awaken frightened almost every night and need extra hugs, comforting, and reassurance. I told her that everything was going to be okay, even though I didn't believe it would be. Every morning I had to fight with my daughter to get her to school. She was afraid to be away from me. I was her best friend and support person. Once I finally got her to the school it made me sick to hear the other mothers in the schoolyard bitching about their problems. If they only knew what real problems were. Boy, to give them the opportunity to step into my shoes for a day. That would sure tune them up in a hurry.

Added to all this was a crummy letter from Sunny Hill, a written assessment which reiterated the diagnosis of attention deficit disorder, severe hyperactivity, and probable autism. The printed words seemed to seal my children's, and my family's, fate. I destroyed the papers before anybody could see them. I didn't even show my husband. I couldn't say the word "autism" for the longest time. I had panic attacks thinking that there was a connection between autism and my little twins. I couldn't accept the fact that my little boys had this disorder. But the hard copy made it real and then, to top it all off, I received a call from Special Services for the Mentally Handicapped, a provincial government agency that offered counselling and programs for families with mentally handicapped children. Mentally handicapped? My boys were mentally handicapped? Now I knew that we had major problems. They must be trying to tell me that my boys are retarded. Funny, this hadn't occurred to me . . . until that phone call.

I remember how the doctor at Sunny Hill told us that the twins might never talk, he couldn't say for sure. No one could predict their potential. I thought at the time that the doctor was a jerk for being so cruel to us. Somehow it made it easier for me to put the blame for my children's handicaps on the doctor that diagnosed them, as if it was his fault. I couldn't think clearly anymore. I started to have more frequent, frightening panic attacks. I didn't know what to do. I even wondered if this was really happening. Maybe it was a huge mistake. How could two of my children be so screwed up?

Well, it was real all right. The papers said so. The doctors said so. And all of the support services that were calling up to offer their assistance were making the message extremely clear.

I remember carrying the twins to bed night after night, thinking, "Are you retarded?" Retarded . . . what is retarded? Oh, yeah, that French word meaning slower, late. Yeah, that's it. They're a little bit slower. Then I would realize that I was trying to downplay the news. We all know what retarded means. It's a cruel word for severely impaired physical or mental function. It's a person who doesn't conform to the norm. A geek, a misfit, a "tard," to quote some of the current slang terms.

I couldn't sleep at night anymore. I would lie awake contemplating different ideas, scenarios, worrying myself sick. Now it didn't matter if the kids woke up; at least it gave me something to do and helped to take my mind off my gloomy thoughts. I couldn't stand to think of what would become of us. What a crappy existence. For all of us.

By the end of October 1991, in an attempt to take control

of our situation, I made a family suicide plan. I decided that if I couldn't go on, I would load up the kids in our van with their favorite blankets and pillows. We would play a game of camping out. We would all cuddle up together, maybe share some special treats, and then, once the kids fell asleep, I would hook the vacuum hose up to the exhaust. Then I would climb back in and hug on to my precious little kids forever. This way they would always be with me. None of us would have to suffer and endure what appeared to be lives of doom. I did not see this as a selfish act but rather an act of pure, unadulterated love, inspired by the maternal instinct to protect my young, to save them from lives which inevitably would be filled with torment, loneliness, and confusion.

Part of what made this whole dilemma so difficult to believe was that Cameron and Brett were good-looking, normal-looking, healthy-looking little three-year-old boys. Physically they were perfect. Mentally, emotionally, they were extremely uptight, agitated, anxious, unhappy, miserable, destructive little brats, but they were *my* little brats and I loved them as much as any mother ever could love her children. It seemed unusual that they would both have the same problem, especially since they were fraternal twins, not identical twins. More than one case of autism in a family is particularly rare. But apparently that's what they had. So what could I do? Learn as much as I could about their diagnosis and try to help these lost little souls.

It was during November 1991 that Judi Langley came into the picture. We were referred to her by Special Services for the Mentally Handicapped, and it was a huge stroke of luck, as Judi got the ball rolling for us.

Judi ran Playcare, a special needs preschool which had a high staff-to-children ratio. This was the only completely segregated preschool remaining in our community — the current educational focus had shifted largely to mainstreaming children with handicaps, but all the children at Playcare had special needs. Children with severe handicaps, such as mine, would never survive in a mainstream situation, a regular preschool, without a lot of behavior interventions and structure. They would not even be accepted into a regular preschool program.

Playcare offered a completely structured program, with one staff member for every two children. It offered a speech and language pathologist once a week. The well-trained staff were experienced at managing children with behavior and language difficulties. They all knew sign language and taught it to the children to increase the number of ways they could communicate (many children with language delay can use sign language much more readily than verbal language). Every few months the staff worked on setting a few realistic goals for each child, accompanied by strategies to attain the goals that would be consistently practised and evaluated for effectiveness in order to find ways to make positive changes in the children's behavior. There was also a focus on education by means of regularly scheduled story time, circle time, arts and crafts, sharing time, etc., that every child attended whether they interacted with the group or not. Everybody was included, everybody was expected to attend each part of the structured session, and this encouraged children to gain appreciation (or at least recognition) of normal classroom structure and routine — something they would all eventually have to be a part of when they were mainstreamed into the regular school system.

Judi was fabulous at her job. She had knowledge, contacts, experience, supportive workers, and a manner that made you feel not so isolated and alone. She never made demands that you were not capable of dealing with. She knew when your energy was running low, helped you get your dignity back, and found ways to help you over the daily hurdles associated with caring for these unusual children. She had a wealth of practical ideas, and it was obvious that families like ours were not new to her. Judi was a lifesaver.

Judi and her assistant Denise started to familiarize them-selves with the twins (and vice versa) by coming into our home once a week for about a month. They would sit on the floor, blow bubbles, pull colorful pictures out of their bags, bring stickers and toys to try to persuade the twins to become interested. My daughter was interested. The twins appeared not to notice. They frequently tried to leave the room. They made no eye contact. There was little interaction. But at least they had all "met," Judi and Denise were now as familiar to the twins as they would ever be — and they could see how difficult it would be to introduce the twins to their pre-school.

But in January 1992 we started taking Cam and Brett into the school for fifteen minutes at a time. The boys were fran-tic, upset, and impossible. They didn't want to go, they screamed and cried when I left the room. Over the course of many months we gradually increased the length of their stay by ten-minute intervals. On several occasions they cried un-til they fell asleep in front of the school door. That's real hard crying. One time one of them tried to climb up on the shelves and get out of a ceiling-level window. The twins were like caged wild animals.

Even getting to school was a problem. As soon as the boys realized that we were headed in the direction of Playcare they would freak out. They would struggle out of their seat belts and try to jump out of the moving vehicle. They would scream, hit, kick, you name it — they did it. I had to drag them in to school on most occasions. They would tear off their clothes and flail on the ground. And because consis-tency is such a large part of modifying the behavior of chil-dren like these, I couldn't give in to their inappropriate reactions. I would repetitively redress them no matter how many times or how long it took, stand them up on their feet (often restraining their arms from hitting me), and direct them in the preschool door. Once they crossed that line I

was free, physically speaking. In my mind the nightmare always continued.

Once inside the doors the twins were the Playcare staff's
responsibility. I felt extremely comfortable with the care the
twins received there. Despite the horrible behavior and difficulties Cam and Brett presented, the staff always handled
the boys with respect, dignity, and patience. Even so, I could
see that the twins were a handful for them. In a way, it was
refreshing to see that other people had as much trouble with
the boys as I did.

As the preschooling progressed to a full morning of activities consisting of three-and-a half hours, I began to get a
bit of a break. I would sit in a small observation booth and
watch through the double-sided mirrored glass as the Playcare staff tried to establish some sense in the twins' bizarre
world of autism. Cam and Brett were clearly very hard to get
through to. They did not want to participate in any of the
activities to begin with. On several occasions they would
dump all of the blocks, puzzle pieces, toys, etc. on the floor
to resist having to participate. The staff member working
with that twin would then have to stop whatever she was
doing, remain calm, sit quietly beside or, in some cases,
physically restrain the twin and, using hand-over-hand technique, begin to pick up each piece until the job was completed. The staff member would have to take my son's hands,
place them on each individual block or puzzle piece one by
one, and place them into the appropriate container or box.
Then appreciative words of encouragement were offered to
the child for completing the job. At first this happened continuously. As the year progressed, it happened less frequently, usually during times of increased frustration and
agitation.

As I watched, Judi would come to sit by me or call me into
her office and offer some excellent tips on how to make our
home life a little easier. She put me in touch with services

that could help to provide a behavior modification program for the twins at home, and she gave me the information to get our children included in a special program designed to help autistic individuals and their families pay for expensive medications and childcare.

Even with all of the extra services now beginning to fall into place, the responsibility of caring for the twins was consuming and depressing. By March 1992 we had our four-year-old twins on a daily double dose of Anafranil. No more Ritalin. They were attending Playcare four mornings a week. Claire, our nanny, had completed her contracted year and let us know that she would be moving on. We couldn't object. God knows we were lucky she stayed with us the whole year. It was a tough one.

As Cam and Brett were finally adapting to school, which gave me a bit of a break, we decided not to hire another nanny. Instead we followed Judi's suggestion that we introduce a childcare worker to the boys at school, and then bring this worker into our home. And so Rosalee entered our lives. Her contract with us was short-lived though, as she made a career change a few months after we met her (nothing personal, I hope).

The next childcare worker to become involved with our twins was Steve Cunningham, a psychology student at Simon Fraser University. He was real easy to look at and had a good sense of humor, was gentle, friendly, sincere, and patient. He liked to have fun and didn't let little things bother him. He had a natural ability to deal with children and a lot of respect for them as people. It amazed me how well he could communicate with kids.

Cameron immediately liked him. When Steve came by for his first interview with me, Cam kept hanging around and was not at all upset about him — an unusual thing to have happen in our household. My boys didn't usually like anyone new that came to our house. So Steve was hired. This proved to be a positive step.

Brett was a little more hesitant to succumb, but he did get along with Steve. Because each child needed constant adult supervision once we stepped out our front door, we soon decided that each boy could benefit more by having his own childcare worker. That way I could spend more time with my daughter and it would provide not only safety for the twins, but also the opportunity for each child to have more individual growth and experiences.

By the time the summer of 1992 rolled around, we had hired another childcare worker, Elizabeth Forrest. Liz, a beautiful redhead, was quiet, softspoken, and very kind and respectful toward the kids. With Elizabeth and Steve, the possibilities really opened up. Before, we had been so limited in what we could do with these unusual children. Now Steve and Liz were taking the twins out of the house twice a week, four hours at a time. What a tremendous break! They worked on keeping the children's clothes on — redressing them each and every time the clothes were removed, even if it took hours. They made sure the twins didn't unbuckle their seatbelts while travelling in the car, even if it meant having to stop every block to rebuckle. They kept a firm grasp on the boys' hands at all times so that the twins could not dash away from the adult and escape. Believe it or not, these were the big goals that we were working on with these little guys. This is what our lives were focusing on. It was pathetic.

Trouble was, nothing made sense to the twins. Language was not coming. Comprehension was almost non-existent, and they could be extremely difficult, especially if they refused their morning dose of Anafranil. The day may as well have ended right then because you knew it would be a disaster if that pill didn't get into them somehow.

As the twins' behavior continued to be bizarre and unacceptable, we were eventually instructed to give, in addition to the Anafranil, three daily doses of Clonidine, another medication which is frequently used for extreme behavioral

problems and agitation. This didn't prove to be very successful, though. We'd spend practically the whole day trying to
trick the boys into taking the medications. We decided we
couldn't live like that so we went back to Anafranil alone.
But now we had a strong group of support people. To finish off the team we decided to hire one more childcare
worker to ensure consistency and to provide backup should
an emergency or difficult period arise. By the end of the summer we hired Kim Pattison.

I knew when I saw the ring in her nose that Kim was right
for the job. To wear that, she had to be very sure of herself.
The rings on her toes said even more. She had an aura of
open-mindedness. She would need to have that to deal with
these strange little kids of mine. With Cam and Brett you
never knew what completely embarrassing thing could happen out in public. You had to have an attitude that said "If
you don't like us it's *your* problem!" Kim definitely had that
attitude. And it was infectious. We all ended up with it.

So we had three wonderful, reliable childcare workers
who were great to the boys and whom the boys were visibly
fond of. They were getting out and doing things. I had more
time to spend with my daughter, sorting out her problems
and getting some activities happening for her. Life was indeed getting a little better.

When the childcare workers had finished their excursions
and the kids were at home again it was disastrous. But each
little break was wonderful. Playcare was slowly giving the
twins some normal routines. It was still hard getting them
to school but at least they were wearing their clothes once
they got there. At home, the stripping never stopped. They
were not going to wear clothes if they had any power in making the decision, and the boys were getting incredibly strong
and quick. It was a day-long job to keep them clothed, and
my husband and I didn't have the stamina to continue the
battle all night, so the clothes stayed off at home.

As the boys grew older, their bizarre behaviors became

worse. Cam and Brett would frequently flap their hands madly and turn around in circles for up to thirty minutes at a time. They were mesmerized by spinning objects. Both boys seemed to need a lot of visual and tactile stimulation. They would watch the TV test pattern or the TV guide channel on our television, but they could not watch a regular TV show. They could not sit for even one page of a book to be read to them, nor could they understand any of it. Their books always had to be torn and shredded. Plates, cups, eggs, bottles, and lightbulbs had to be smashed. They were completely mesmerized by the way the shards of glass scattered on the floor. I think they found the sound of imploding glass very stimulating, too.

Even with the small improvement produced by the Anafranil, the twins could not stand any type of orderliness in the house. They always tipped our chairs upside down. Every time I picked them back up, they would knock them down again. Their toys had to be scattered around the house. Whenever they were put into a toybox, the twins would pull them back out again and throw them around. Same thing with food, it had to be crushed and scattered around the house. Sitting at the dinner table for a meal was absolutely out of the question. They were not capable of sitting for any length of time, nor were they interested in eating a meal. There weren't many foods they would eat. Instead, they chewed little chunks of the drywall in our house and bit pieces of the interior panels of our van. They put anything they could find into their mouths — so long as it wasn't food. And as I've said, they had a real problem with toileting; everything had to be smeared all around the house.

Out in the back yard the scattering continued. The twins would pull bedding plants out of the garden and throw them on the lawn. They put handfuls of newspaper and dirt into the hot tub. Brett managed to pull down a pile of stacked 6" x 6" landscaping ties one time to break the orderliness. Unfortunately, one fell on his foot and broke it. But Brett felt no pain. He cried for a few minutes and then was back pulling more ties down. We took him to the local North Vancouver hospital for an x-ray that showed the foot was definitely broken. The doctor thought there was no point in putting a cast on as Brett would clearly not tolerate it. We agreed.

By the next morning Brett was hopping, running, and doing his circles again despite the broken foot. We were amazed and took him to Children's Hospital in Vancouver to have the foot x-rayed again. The x-ray showed a broken foot alright.

Another example of the twins' utter disregard for safety is an incident from December 1991. We had a string of Christmas lights up around the edge of our upstairs balcony because the boys would put the lights in their mouths and bite them if they were on the Christmas tree — even if they were lit up. One of the twins (I can't remember which one it was now) climbed right over the railings to put the lights in his mouth. Luckily he had a firm grasp of the lightbulb because he lost his footing and fell. It was like a scene from *Raiders of the Lost Ark*. He came streaming down to the family-room floor hanging on to a strand of lights, got up, and then tried to do it again.

Then there was the time that Brett caught my daughter's goldfish in his hands and squished its guts out. And the time he sprayed our kitchen floor with non-stick spray and went ice skating on it. Incidentally, so did I. I had no idea what he had done, so when I stepped onto the kitchen floor I took a dive. Was I pissed off! But what a neat idea.

When they weren't spinning and smashing things, they would sit on a couch in front of a window and stare out into space. If you tried to get in front of them to make eye contact, they would pull a book up in front of their face and block you out. There was no getting in to their private isolation.

There were also some things that the twins could do well.

They call these splinter skills. Cameron could run the TV, VCR, stereo, and compact disc player by himself. Even my daughter and husband had trouble doing these things. When I bought a computer, Cameron set up the screen, typed in the menu code, and started playing games. He knew how to operate most of the programs before I had a chance to read the manuals. By watching him we learned how to use the computer programs. Then there was the time he got the keys and started the van. When he went to put it into gear we got a little worried. I'm sure this kid thought that he could drive.

The boys had a keen sense of smell. When the childcare workers or any relatives came to the house, the boys would smell their car keys; they knew what belonged to who through a sense of smell. They paid particular attention to the smell of clothing, and at preschool they were often observed smelling the other children.

They also had a keen sense of direction. So keen, in fact, that when out driving, if we dared to take a wrong turn (that is, a turn that Cam and Brett weren't expecting us to take) all hell would break loose. We would have to backtrack and turn in exactly the "right" direction. They knew where every McDonald's was in the city. And unfortunately, and perhaps because of the dependency upon consistency and structure that we were trying to instill into these guys, because we would sometimes go to a McDonald's drive-through we now had to go into every McDonald's drive-through that we passed or else the guys would become agitated and confused, screaming and upset for the rest of the day. If the twins didn't get exactly what they wanted, if their schedule was changed or expectations were not met, the result was chaos. But they couldn't talk, they couldn't answer yes or no to a question, they couldn't understand the question in the first place, or tell us what they were expecting, so we were never sure what wrong turn or deviation from the norm had set them off.

And then there was this ever-present disrobing. They didn't understand the need to wear clothes at all. It didn't matter how cold it was — Cameron and Brett didn't seem to feel the cold. The sooner they could get their clothes off, the better. And once they were off, it was difficult to convince them to put the clothing back on. Their thought patterns were so primitive. So were their responses.

So there they were, no meaningful verbal language skills, almost no comprehension of language, extremely strange mannerisms, behavior, and sense of smell, sight, and sensation. All pointing in the direction of autism. What a job we had ahead of us.

3

The Birth of a Miracle

September 23, 1992. At first, it appeared to be another humungous piece of bad luck, a case of being in the wrong place at the wrong time.

One of our childcare workers, Elizabeth, had agreed to babysit for us on Wednesday nights, so my husband and I were finally able to go out "dating" again without having to worry about the safety of the kids. We were on our way out to dinner this night, waiting for a light to change at the bottom of a steep hill, when we were rear-ended in our van and punched clear across to the other side of the intersection. In two seconds I got a double-whammy of significant whiplash and jaw problems.

This accident was to be the best thing that could have happened to me. But not right away. For the next four months I was in constant pain with neck and back spasms. I had appointments galore. Physiotherapy, massage therapy, insurance company appointments, doctor's appointments, preschool and childcare appointments. After the initial four months there were also pain clinic, biofeedback, and dentist appointments. I spent the majority of my "spare time" lying on ice packs for pain relief. I was on narcotics for many months. I was becoming very depressed about the way things were going.

Our family life deteriorated further and our twins started to regress. We couldn't focus as much time and attention on their behavior programs. I couldn't really look after the kids but I still had to. There was little I could do except let them run around and do their thing. It was difficult for me to dress them, lift them, pull them off cupboards, etc. And it was particularly painful when they resisted my attempts to physically restrain them. My neck ached, my head ached, my back ached, and my jaws were killing me. I was having a terrible time trying to cope.

They did unbelievable things. For example, they poured a whole bottle of ketchup on the kitchen floor, skated through it in bare feet, and then ran to get away from me, spreading ketchup all over the house. It looked as though a gruesome murder had occurred in our home. They would defecate on their bedroom floor and then jump into it and run through the house. They spilled eight litres of milk on the kitchen floor and attempted to swim in it. These were big messes to clean — especially as I was in such pain. And I struggled to keep my temper controlled. I always consider these kids to be lucky; if I had child-beating tendencies, these little guys would have been toast.

Every morning was a two-hour effort to get the twins out of bed, get them medicated, get them fed, and somehow get them out the door to school, preferably with their clothes on. Several times I had to throw all of the clothes in the van, wrestle the kids in, and drive them to school naked. With any luck, by the time I got into the Playcare parking lot they would finally obey and get dressed. There were, however, a couple of times when I had no choice but to bring them in half clad. I hated getting my daughter to school late all the time. I hated the anxiety and agitation, the screaming and crying every morning.

When I tried to carry out our behavior modification program the boys would jump on my back, pull my hair, yank my arms, kick, yell, bite. More often than not, I would have to pick them up and physically restrain them to maintain control until the moment of particularly bizarre behavior had passed.

The twins yelled, screamed, roared like monsters, and made all kinds of weird, inappropriate sounds. They spun in circles and flapped their hands like seals' flippers. I kept trying to imagine where they were at, what was going on in their minds. How was I ever going to get through to them? Why couldn't they see the pattern of normal social interactions? Why didn't anything make sense to them? What were we going to do with them? And what would happen to them? Group homes? Or would they live with us forever? I guessed they would. I guessed that I would be their lifelong babysitter, provider, advocate, mother, housemaid.

I knew that I had to get over my injury quickly so that I could regain control, but after five months I was getting frustrated with my lack of recovery. My neck and jaw problems were getting worse, not better. I was finally referred to a new doctor who was highly recommended by my massage therapist. She said that he had special interest and training in the assessment and treatment of soft-tissue injuries. She made the first appointment for me while I was in her office. I was to see Dr. Zigurts Strauts for the first time on February 15, 1993.

Zigurts had an office across town from where I lived. At one point my pain was so severe, and the drive was so long, I considered cancelling the appointment. Luckily, I reconsidered.

When I arrived for the appointment, the doctor began by asking for my basic past health history, for an account of the car accident that I was in, and then for my family profile. When I mentioned that I had two autistic children he suddenly stopped writing and looked right into my eyes. He asked what their symptoms were. I told him that my two little boys, who were now almost five years old, were extremely anxious and agitated. They were, in fact, quite demented. They were hyperactive, couldn't speak much, and couldn't tell you what their names were if you asked. They also destroyed practically everything that we owned. They were obnoxious and destructive. Why, they even ate the walls.

"They ate the walls?" he asked, still looking into my eyes.

"Yes, they bit chunks out of the drywall and they bit chunks out of the inside of our van in some places."

"Did anyone ever test them for allergies or sensitivities?"

"Not really. The twins don't cooperate well enough for any doctor to assess them," I stated.

"Do you live near any highways?" he asked.

"We lived on Mountain Highway for the twins' first couple years of life."

"You mean right beside the highway?" he asked.

"Yes."

"Was your home old or new?"

"It wasn't very old. It was built in the early seventies, I think."

"Did you do any remodelling or painting?" he asked.

"Tons of it. We had two sundecks built, the whole house painted inside and out. We had a couple of sections of walls removed and quite a few changes in bathroom fixtures and plumbing. But why does this matter?" I asked.

"Hmm . . . they ate the walls . . . uphill car emissions . . . renovations . . . Did anyone ever test them for lead or other heavy metals? Or trace minerals?" he asked.

"No."

"I think they may be suffering from lead poisoning," he said.

What was this guy talking about? Cameron and Brett's behavior was so severely affected that such a quick deduction, a simple solution like this didn't seem possible. And how would they have been poisoned anyhow? Nobody else had ever mentioned this possibility.

"No, I really mean it," he said, obviously reading my reaction. "It sounds like they may be lead or mercury poisoned. We've got to check them out."

I don't remember anything more about the visit. What I

do remember is nearly having another car accident on the way home. I couldn't stop thinking about what Zigurts had said. On the one hand, I wanted to believe that it could be true. At least lead or mercury poisoning is treatable. But on the other hand, it's so hard to set yourself up for failure and disappointment when you have kids like this. They'd already seen a multitude of the best doctors in town and nobody else had ever suspected this.

But . . . what if he was right?

I went right from my appointment with Zigurts to a meeting with the preschool teachers and childcare workers at Playcare. We were to discuss current issues and future goals, evaluate the previous set of goals and strategies, and discuss whether our current interventions were working.

I blew in the door flustered and excited by what had transpired at the doctor's office. I described Zigurts' reaction to the boys' diagnosis of autism and his thoughts about their condition. The team members listened patiently, then said "That's interesting," and wanted to get started on the day's topics. My bubble was burst. I knew that I was getting my hopes up. Of course metal poisoning was too simple an explanation for the complex disorder my twins had. The team was right. Time to get back down to the nitty gritty of planning goals and strategies and measuring their slow progress to date.

During the week before my next appointment with Zigurts my husband asked his co-workers at Children's Hospital about the possibility that the twins could have picked up excessive heavy metals, namely lead. The response was not favorable. Most of the pediatricians said that it was a shot in the dark. The lab technicians' best advice was "Kids don't have lead poisoning around here. You only find that in the ghetto areas in the United States or lead smelter towns like Trail [a town in the interior of British Columbia]." No one gave the idea any credibility. And these people worked with children all the time.

At this point, though, there is one thing that I should tell you about myself. I have this motto — this attitude . . . Never leave any stone unturned. Thank God I had that motto. And thank God Zigurts had the knowledge and good sense to believe in himself. It was hard to get too excited about the whole thing, though. You can imagine how difficult it is to feel optimistic when professional people are telling you that you are wasting your time, that you're looking for answers that aren't there.

At my next appointment, Zigurts breezed through my chart and then asked, "Remember what I said about your kids?"

"Well, yes," I said. "As a matter of fact, I haven't thought of anything else. Do you really think that this could be a possibility? Everyone else we've talked to thinks that we're desperate and are looking for a miracle. They say that this could never happen here."

"That's because they have a lack of knowledge in this area. A couple of years ago I wouldn't have looked for this either. Heavy metals are an area of special interest and knowledge to me, though I usually work with adults."

He seemed very confident about testing the twins for lead and other heavy metals. And what the heck, we had nothing to lose. So Zigurts asked me to bring in my twins.

As you can guess, kids like mine you don't just "bring in." Getting them out the front door is close to impossible on a good day, but to take the two of them in to wait and perform at a doctor's office . . . The twins would tear the place to pieces. I told the doctor that I would bring one in at a time. It would be plenty of hard work to accomplish that. He responded with, "Okay, Nancy, if that's all you feel you can handle." There it was again! Nobody ever believed how difficult my two little children could be. I winced knowing that he was thinking maybe it was Mrs. Hallaway who had the problem and not her boys. He would change his mind when he met them. That I knew for sure. I was nervous that, once the doctor saw them, he would realize that the twins' condition was much worse than he thought, that by the end of the appointment he would tell me he had made a mistake.

When the day came for Brett's appointment with Zigurts I made sure that I had a bag full of "ammunition" — books, toys, gum, everything I could think of that might get us through the appointment with as few problems as possible. I had to get the Playcare staff to sneak Brett out of the classroom without his brother noticing because that would have been sure to set off panic for them both.

The drive across town to the office went well but, once there, Brett spotted a coffee shop with huge, gooey, iced cinnamon buns in the front window. The visit came to a halt while Brett had his first tantrum on busy Granville Street. I was nervous and embarrassed. To avoid a bigger scene, in we went to buy a bun. What a mess. There was icing and cinnamon all over his hands and clothes. This I hadn't come prepared for.

The wait in the office seemed to last a week. I had trouble keeping Brett in the reception room. I could see other patients looking at me with expressions that said, "Can't you control that child?" The truth was, I was doing an incredibly fine job of controlling this impossible child. If others could only step into my shoes and dance to the music that I had to.

Brett spotted something that intrigued him in another office and there was no stopping his attempts to get in there. When I pulled him out and dragged him back to Zigurts' office, he had a second tantrum in the hallway. Brett was screaming, kicking, biting. My temper was starting to flare up, I felt that familiar headache coming on, and my teeth were clenching.

Finally we went in to see the doctor. Brett was a disaster. Zigurts realized that there was no point in trying to physically examine Brett. He was far too aggressive and agitated, and confused about what was going on. I could tell by the look on the doctor's face that this behavior was worse than he'd expected.

Luckily, Zigurts and I had an excellent rapport. He made it clear that he felt sorry for kids like this. He was a father of four children himself and had a good grasp of the difficulty raising even typical children. He was aware that kids with behavior problems were the ones that ended up the losers, the dropouts, the criminals, or the vulnerable, abused people of society.

Because it was practically impossible to do anything but manage Brett while the appointment took place, the doctor asked me to come back alone the next day so we could discuss testing for the twins. Discuss testing. That meant he really did think there was a chance my kids were lead poisoned. I was flying.

The drive home with Brett was also a disaster but it didn't matter to me. I was fantasizing about what it would be like to have my two little boys become "normal." I knew that it was still a longshot, but I could dream. That was something that could never be taken away from me. And I knew that I could still live with the twins the way they were if this turned out to be a wild goose chase.

That night I could hardly sleep. I couldn't wait to get to the doctor's office to get the information and begin testing for lead. Just having something definite to test for was a great feeling, even if the results might not turn out the way we hoped. Disorders such as autism, attention deficit disorder, and hyperactivity have no definitive tests. There are many different traits to look for and behaviors which are suggestive of these disorders. But no test can tell you either yes or no, your child is autistic or not. Diagnoses of these disorders are based on professional opinions about symptoms a child shows, and the symptoms of these associated disorders vary from child to child. Some symptoms are present in one case and not in another, or one symptom disappears while others pop up. They are such abstract diagnoses to live with, and there is often no definitive reason why the symptoms or disorders occur. There are theories. Sometimes allergies are to blame, or diet. Some people suggest that a change in diet helps. Some think that parenting is the real problem while others figure that these kids may have been affected by a virus during pregnancy. Many speculate that genetics are responsible. Many physicians think it could be a combination of these factors. The causes and the diagnoses are all vague and subjective.

When I went in for the next appointment I was afraid Zigurts might think I was becoming too convinced that metal poisoning was the answer. I was again very nervous. I wanted to assure him that I could face the outcome of the testing, even if it was negative. I didn't want him to think that he might be getting my hopes up too high. Maybe then he would change his mind about testing my twins, perhaps thinking that he was offering false hope.

But Zigurts didn't waver. He knew that the boys should be tested. In fact, he felt that it was unreasonable not to test them for heavy metals. He was so confident. He trusted his judgment. And so did I. As a nurse, I had a real good gut feeling that he was looking at these children's best interests.

And so we discussed the importance of testing for body burden, the quantity of lead and other metals that has accumulated in body tissues. (I've tried to keep medical terms and jargon to a minimum, but sometimes I can't avoid them. Refer to the glossary at the end of the book for definitions of unfamiliar words.) He carefully explained when and how to test, and gave me the specimen containers for the tests. I was instructed to get a hair sample from each twin, and a special urine sample after giving the boys Cuprimine, a chelating agent that would pull metal ions from their body tissues. I knew that getting these samples would not be a problem. The problem would come later when I tried to get the twins to *stop* peeing in the cup. I left feeling happy and confident about what we were about to do. (For a full description of chelation treatment and how it works, see Chapter 6.)

I went to the drug store immediately to fill the prescription. The pharmacist was startled that I would be giving this medication to a child. "This is for arthritis," she said. I knew that. But I knew that it was also for deleading body tissues. So she filled the prescription and I took it home.

We started the Cuprimine on a weekend so that the boys could get all of the doses at the proper intervals. Cuprimine (alias penicillamine) stinks! It tastes bad and smells terrible. Getting kids to swallow this is not easy. It is in the form of a capsule which is too big for a small child to swallow, so I had to mix the medicine with a small quantity of water or juice, put it into a syringe, hold each boy in a half-nelson, and plunge the syringe into their mouths. My technique didn't always work as I had hoped, but getting any of it into them would give us some results if there were any to be found. I must admit, the hair sample was much easier.

A few days later I returned to the doctor's office with my little samples, and entrusted them to the nurse's hands. They were like precious gold to me. I wanted them to be well taken care of. I wanted the results even more. And I'll tell you why I wanted them so badly. I had started to do a little research of my own about metal poisoning, and what I was reading astounded me. I had the feeling that Zigurts was absolutely right.

After the three-day dose of Cuprimine, the change in the twins' behavior and disposition was unbelievable. It was obvious to all who had direct contact with my twin boys. Their agitation and anxiety significantly decreased. Every morning their cute little faces would poke out of their covers and display huge smiles. They were sleeping well for a change. They hopped out of bed and happily got ready (with help) for school. They let me put their clothes on. Then they marched out of the door to the van like soldiers. They didn't mind going to school anymore. And once there, no more kicking, biting, or fighting. They grabbed their respective articles and marched in to the classroom. We even made it to school on time on most occasions now. This had never happened before.

By April 7, 1993, my children's specimens had been gone for three weeks. My phone rang at four o'clock in the afternoon. I picked it up and said, "Hello."

"Hello, happy lady!" said the confident, deep voice on the other end of the line.

"Am I happy?" was my response. I had no idea who it was or what this call was about.

"You sure are happy," said the mysterious voice.

I thought I recognized the voice but couldn't place it — or maybe it was a telephone salesperson or a wrong number. "Who am I speaking to?"

"Dr. Strauts," he said.

I just about fell on the floor. Now I knew exactly what this call was about. And he said "happy lady," right? He must have some good news. "What were the results?"

"Your two little boys appear to have a problem with elevated lead and arsenic. Their lead level is about three times higher than the acceptable level. Cameron also has elevated cadmium levels." I knew from the investigating I had been doing that cadmium was extremely toxic to the developing child — perhaps more toxic than lead.

A huge weight lifted off my shoulders. My little boys were probably not autistic at all. They were poisoned, and metal poisoning can be treated.

"Come in and see me tomorrow," Zigurts said.

I couldn't even hear anymore! The blood seemed to be rushing through my body and I was feeling lightheaded. This must be what they call an adrenalin rush. I felt like I had won a multimillion-dollar lottery. And what incredible luck that I had connected with Zigurts in the first place.

When my feet touched the ground again, and I got in to the office, I saw the test results which made it clear my little twins were indeed severely metal poisoned. The remarkable change in their behavior reinforced these results. Now we had a whole new angle, something concrete we could work with. We still had no idea how much or how successful a recovery the twins would make. No one would ever be able to measure what their intended potential was. But we had hope, perhaps more than hope. From the difference of the last few weeks, I knew that the improvements were happening, dramatically and rapidly.

We started treatment by giving Cam and Brett trace mineral supplements. Not only were the boys showing toxic amounts of heavy metals, they also exhibited deficiencies in such trace minerals as silicon, lithium, strontium, and vanadium. These deficiencies are often encountered in lead-toxic individuals, and the minerals must be restored as they could be further depleted by the next course of chelation therapy.

Then our children were treated with another course of Cuprimine. Within one week of the treatment, Cameron and Brett were showing more astounding improvement. They were happy and affectionate almost all of the time. One of the twins actually said to me, "I happy!" These little guys were finally beginning to talk. They were beginning to use real, meaningful words. They were obviously impressed with their new abilities. And they had no further problems with separation anxiety. They let me out of their sight willingly. They even encouraged me to go out on several occasions. They were becoming self-confident and comfortable without me.

Cameron and Brett started to "pink up." Previously their facial coloring had been pasty and pale. They always seemed to have dark circles under their eyes. We thought that they were chronically tired-looking because their sleeping habits were so poor, but now their color dramatically improved — they began to look pink and healthy. Their hands and feet, which previously were always cold — like little blocks of ice — became warm and pink, too. It was obvious that they had been anemic — another symptom of lead toxicity. Why no one had ever noticed this before is beyond me but then, I had never given it any thought, either.

Cameron and Brett had always displayed strange sleeping habits, with frequent tremors and twitching. My husband and I used to wonder if this was a relatively mild form of seizure activity. It certainly was not the usual movement of REM (rapid eye movement) sleep or vivid dream activity. However, after the second treatment they no longer twitched or jerked while sleeping.

By day they were active but not hyperactive. They used much less energy performing unnecessary body movements, and had a reasonable attention span. They could focus on activities with very little prompting for longer periods of time. They could stay on task with less effort. And their eye contact . . . what a change! Now they could tune in and focus on our faces, actually look into our eyes.

Since the day that Zigurts called me with the greatest news of my life, there never passes a moment in which I don't feel like the luckiest lady on earth. My family has a new lease on life. What always goes through my mind is my daughter's little request, her innocent wish that one day the boys would be able to talk and play with her. Do you believe in miracles? I do now. My daughter's wish is going to be answered.

1

Are We Ready
to Accept the Evidence?

As my children were in the process of metal detoxification
I continued to do my own research on the subject of metal
poisoning. One of the studies I found, carried out by Debo-
rah Rice and R.F. Willes of the Health Protection Branch of
Health and Welfare Canada in 1979, amazed me. It involved
two groups of monkeys. Because brain development in monkeys and people is similar, monkeys are often used for research into neurological development. In Rice and Willes'
study, a group of monkeys was exposed to constant low levels of lead from birth to age three. They showed a blood lead
level similar to levels that were being observed in most Canadian children during that period of time. These levels were
not believed at that time to produce intellectual and behavioral disorders, but by the third year the monkeys exhibited
all of the behaviors that my twin boys exhibited. These monkeys were much more active than untreated monkeys. They
were, in fact, hyperactive. Their ability to inhibit unwanted
responses or to control their behavior was retarded, as was
their ability to adapt easily to demands placed upon them.
They behaved inconsistently from day to day, even minute
to minute. They had attention and memory problems and
their ability to learn was impaired. They were impulsive. I
would bet my last dollar that if they could have been tested
for language development they probably would have been
language delayed — just like my boys.

I might have been reading about Cam and Brett. It was obvious to me that there was a connection between lead's effects on these monkeys and what had been happening to my kids. There have been enough other studies carried out on both children and laboratory animals in the past 30 years to show that too much exposure to lead and other metals causes increased distractibility, decreased organizational skills, inability to follow simple and complex instructions, and low overall functioning in a classroom setting. Research shows that, during school years, lead-exposed children exhibit behavioral problems, lower IQ, and deficiencies in speech and language comprehension — and teenagers with histories of lead exposure drop out of school seven times as often as their peers.

Why didn't anyone put two and two together and suggest we test Cam and Brett? One thing that became obvious to me as I talked about metal poisoning with other parents, my kids' teachers and workers, and professional colleagues (laboratory technicians, doctors, health officials, nurses, etc.) is that everyone believes it is no longer a problem. Because lead has been removed from paint and gasoline, the feeling is that kids are no longer affected, or that it's only a problem in developing countries or run-down inner cities. But lead is still in paint on the walls of many houses built before the 1980s, lead and other metals are in the soil, in our water, and in many other places we don't suspect (see Chapter 9 to find out "Where Is the Stuff Coming From?").

Metals are often not recognized as a problem because blood test results do not indicate long-term low-level exposure, only recent short-term exposure. The body burden of lead (the lead that has accumulated in body tissues) cannot be determined with any accuracy by a blood test because the lead only stays in the bloodstream for a few weeks. Other metals that can damage a child's developing nervous system, either alone or in combination with lead, are not generally screened for in a blood sample. It is important to be aware that, although a child might not show a significantly high blood lead level in a random blood sample, he may in fact be carrying a huge amount of lead or other metals in his body if he has been exposed to a consistent low level of lead and other metals every day of his early developing life.

By the way, I purposely use the male pronoun here. For some reason boys are more susceptible to metal poisoning than girls are. A recent study from Hamilton's McMaster University indicates that women have denser brain tissue than men. Women have 11 percent more nerve cells in the areas of the brain (including the hippocampus, the amygdala, and the cerebral cortex) that process speech and language, which are also the areas often affected by metal poisoning. Because women have more nerve cells to "spare" they may have an increased ability to function in spite of damage to the brain. Another theory suggests that girls tend to house more toxic metals in fat cells of the body than do males. Perhaps it is a hormonally controlled phenomenon. At any rate, it is an area that bears some further investigation.

Ironically, as the general public dismisses metal poisoning as a disease of the past, researchers have been lowering the accepted level for blood lead in the human body, recognizing that metals have toxic effects at lower levels than was previously believed, on children in particular. Researchers are also recognizing that other metals can be more toxic than lead. In 1970 a blood reading over 60 micrograms (µg) of lead per decilitre (dl) of blood was considered toxic. This level was decreased to 25 µg/dl in 1988 and to 10 µg/dl in 1991. And now researchers have found a definite reduction of IQ in children with a blood lead level of less than 10 µg/dl. In 1992 the Centers for Disease Control (CDC) and the Environmental Protection Agency (EPA) in the United States estimated that one out of every six American children — as many as 4 million — had high lead levels (10 µg/dl and higher), levels that researchers have shown to be responsible for detectable neurological damage (*i.e.*, learning disabilities, decreased growth, hyperactivity, impaired hearing, brain damage).

This reduction in what were previously considered to be safe levels of lead in the blood does not mean that the effects of lead have suddenly become worse. Rather, it's a result of increasingly sensitive measuring techniques that allow researchers to detect levels of lead and other metals in body tissues, and to make the connection between neurological damage and the presence of even small quantities of metals that could cause it.

The level at which lead should be considered toxic has been a hotly debated issue for the last two decades. Back in the early 1970s, three doctors at Harvard Medical School began studying the effects of an increased lead burden in children. In October 1972, Siegfried Pueschel and his colleagues Louis Kopito and Harry Schwachman published "Children With an Increased Lead Burden — A Screening and Follow-up Study" in the *Journal of the American Medical Association*. Pueschel released another study, "Neurological and Psychomotor Functions in Children with an Increased Lead Burden," in May 1974's *Environmental Health Perspectives*. They reported that, in many cases, children with an increased lead burden did not show major signs or symptoms, so they escaped medical attention. Pueschel, Kopito, and Schwachman found that in cases of mild or subacute toxicity, the symptoms were often vague or nonspecific, sometimes even non-existent. In many cases children complained of symptoms like abdominal pain, diarrhea, vomiting, constipation, loss of appetite, clumsiness, irritability, increase in sleepiness, drowsiness, convulsions, and/or headaches. The Harvard team emphasized that, particularly in cases where young children with obvious neurological and gastro-intestinal problems also have a history of "pica" (eating non-food substances such as paint, dirt, rocks, crayons, etc.), there should be a strong suspicion of lead toxicity.

They stated that the need for early recognition of children

with an increased lead burden was crucial since failure to identify them could leave them susceptible to mental retardation and developmental delay. When children who tested positive for lead poisoning were given appropriate treatment, and when environmental hazards were eliminated, serious damage to the central nervous system could be prevented. The children showed a significant gain in IQ points when they were treated with chelating agents for deleading body tissues. However, permanent nervous system damage was still often observed during follow-up examinations of previously lead-poisoned children despite the deleading procedure.

In conclusion, the Harvard group found that, where initial assessments of these children showed low average mental abilities, follow-up assessments made eighteen months to three years later showed a significant increase in certain areas of intellectual functioning. This was a comprehensive, detailed study, and the results clearly support the need for early testing and diagnosis to prevent the occurrence of gross neurological damage in children. Furthermore, they support the need to test for lead toxicity in those children already experiencing neurological dysfunction, as treatment can still produce measurable improvement.

The Harvard group described kidney problems in later life as another possible consequence of long-term lead toxicity. In their studies they found that patients with a previous history of lead poisoning had albuminuria (protein), glycosuria (sugar), and other abnormal findings in their urine. Other studies have indicated abnormal findings in the initial stages of lead poisoning — urine samples of lead-toxic children have shown early signs of kidney tissue disturbance.

Five years after the Harvard study, research conducted at McGill University in 1977 suggested a new method of testing for metal body burden that can help catch metal-toxic children who aren't showing obvious symptoms. "Hair Elemental Content in Learning Disabled Children" presented a significant relationship between lead and other heavy metal content in hair, and the presence of learning disabilities in children. R.O. Pihl and M. Parkes of the Department of Psychology at McGill University conducted a study on a group of 53 children: 31 children were learning-disabled while 22 were "typical" children. Pihl and Parkes found that they could separate the two groups by analyzing hair samples for fourteen heavy metals.

The learning-disabled children in this study exhibited a range of disabilities in the areas of hearing, spoken language, orientation, behavior, and motor skills. Severely mentally handicapped and neurologically impaired children were excluded from this study so the group displayed a good random selection of children from a typical school setting.

The hair was collected from the children according to laboratory procedures and analyzed by atomic absorption spectroscopy. Analysis of the fourteen elements yielded definite differences between the two groups of children. Elevated levels of any metals were noted, but Pihl and Parkes found a strong, negative correlation between lead and cobalt (the learning disabled children had an excess of lead and a deficiency of cobalt) and a positive correlation between lead and cadmium (there was an excess of both lead and cadmium in learning disabled children). The summary of the study indicated that, using measurements of lead, cadmium, cobalt, manganese, chromium, and lithium in hair, subjects could be classified as learning disabled or normal with 98 percent accuracy. This result was unexpected.

The report also concluded that, although the learning disabled children's hair samples showed lower amounts of metal than were considered toxic, the evidence suggested that exposure to low concentrations of metals has detrimental effects on behavior. Pihl and Parkes mentioned childhood hyperactivity as one syndrome gaining considerable attention in this regard, and emphasized that their research, as well as other studies, suggest that hair analysis may be a useful diagnostic procedure which could relate lead and metal toxicity to the cause of specific disorders

In 1986 the Royal Society of Canada's Commission on Lead in the Environment produced a report, *The Health Effects of Lead*, which summarized much of the research into lead poisoning. As in the McGill and Harvard studies, diagnosis of lead poisoning was a major issue. The extensive Royal Society report indicated that, in studies of children with increased lead burden, blood lead levels failed to show a significant correlation to body burden of lead and other metals. In other words, a blood lead level may show only a slight measurement of lead whereas more extensive testing (for example hair elemental analysis or urine testing with chelation challenge) may reveal a large amount of lead that has been sequestered in the body tissues and bones. There can be huge discrepancies in test results between these methods. As lead stays in the blood for only a short time, a random blood sample for lead is not a good measurement for revealing chronic lead toxicity. The Royal Society concluded that blood levels were good indicators of recent exposure to lead but were very poor indicators of the body burden of lead, and that a more sophisticated method for measuring the body burden of lead is essential. This is an extremely critical piece of information to bear in mind when testing for lead in the neurologically impaired child.

The Royal Society's report also acknowledged that lead metabolism in infants and young children places them in far higher risk categories than older humans (this is discussed in more detail in Chapter 5), and revealed that many Canadian infants are commonly exposed to dietary intakes of lead which exceed the acceptable levels. It stated that the average Canadian infant consumes five times the average intake of lead for all age groups. The report said that, as some of the more subtle toxicological effects of lead are only now being understood, it is vital that steps be taken as quickly as possible to reduce infants' exposure to lead from food and environmental sources. The research indicated that exposure levels previously considered to be safe caused definite changes in behavior, and recent evidence points to the fact that relatively low body burdens of lead can result in lower IQ in children. This finding is consistent with the impaired learning ability observed in animals tested both in the Royal Society's studies and others.

Holly Ruff and Polly Bijur of the Divisions of Behavioral Paediatrics and Epidemiology at Albert Einstein College of Medicine reported on their research in a 1989 article "The Effects of Low to Moderate Lead Levels on Neurobehavioral Functioning in Children." They stated that the absorption of low to moderate levels of lead results in the storage of lead in the brain. Small amounts of lead can disrupt both brain morphology (form or structure of the anatomy) and physiology (functioning of component parts). In analyzing brain tissue after death, they found significant changes in some areas of the brain. More lead accumulated in the hippocampus, the amygdala, and the cerebral cortex than in other parts of the brain. These three areas are largely responsible for behavior, emotions, and language/speech.

Ruff and Bijur suggest that even low lead levels may result in fewer and less mature synapses in the brain. Lead also interferes with neurotransmitter function and causes disruption of normal cellular activity. This is what's believed to cause the neurological impairment. And don't forget, we're talking about low levels of lead here. Other studies have already confirmed that high levels of lead cause disease of the peripheral nerves in animals and humans, and large amounts of lead can demyelinate motor nerves — destroying the nerves' protective covering. Ruff and Bijur are making the point that this damage can occur when lead is present at much lower levels than previously thought.

The Einstein College team also found that there was a strong relationship between lead and cadmium in that they almost always show up together. They suggested it is possible that cadmium acts independently on the nervous system and compounds the devastation of lead toxicity by causing, by itself, extreme nervous system damage. They also found evidence to support the fact that there is an interaction between lead intake and nutrition: deficiencies of either calcium or iron seem to enhance the detrimental effects of lead, whereas an abundance of either element seems to prevent lead absorption.

Ruff and Bijur indicated that better assessments of body burden must be performed to fully understand the harmful effects of lead on children. They recognized that a simple blood test is inadequate to produce a conclusive measure of body burden or chronic lead exposure and toxicity. Blood lead reflects recent exposure, but other measures are needed to reflect the amount of lead in soft tissues and bone. They were hopeful that recent developments in x-ray fluorescence (a method for detecting the amount of lead sequestered in the bones) might prove it to be the simplest and most practical method for accurately measuring the body burden of lead. Unfortunately, this test is not readily available in the U.S., and is not offered at all in Canada yet.

Holly Ruff also presented some optimistic findings about the reversibility of moderate lead poisoning in an April 1993 study in the *Journal of the American Medical Association*. Ruff and her fellow researchers from Albert Einstein College of Medicine found that for each 3 µg/dl that blood levels were decreased, there was a one-point increase in a cognitive index scale derived from standardized intelligence tests. The mean blood lead levels of children in the study fell from 31.2 to 23.9 µg/dl and their mean cognitive index scores rose from 79 to 82.6. The children in the study ranged in age from seven to thirteen, by which time most brain growth has already occurred, so the fact that detoxification produced improvements is encouraging for parents of older children.

Blood lead levels of 23.9 µg/dl are still excessive, and since no measure of accumulated body burden was given, my assumption is that most of these children had very high levels of accumulated lead. Rather than being moderately toxic, they may have been severely toxic and would therefore require continued chelation until the blood levels and tissue levels of accumulated lead dropped to more acceptable levels. Such a drop may cause another rise in cognitive index scores.

After reading all these reports and studies I turned to the *Diagnostic and Statistical Manual of Mental Disorders* (DSM-III-R), the American Psychiatric Association's handbook for diagnosing mental handicaps, which clearly recognizes lead as a possible causative factor for mental retardation. Among the disorders, syndromes, and other "labels" for which the DSM-III-R cites lead and other metals as possible causes are: pervasive developmental disorder, borderline intellectual functioning, mild mental retardation, moderate mental retardation, severe mental retardation, profound mental retardation, unspecified mental retardation, autistic disorder, and academic skills disorder. The criteria used to measure and assess such disorders in children focus on the inadequate development of academic, language, speech, and motor skills. The manual lists symptoms of mental retardation and some of the other disorders as including passivity, dependency, low self-esteem, low frustration tolerance, aggressiveness, poor impulse control, self-stimulating behavior, and self-injurious behavior.

In light of all of these well-documented studies, academic research, and medical knowledge indicating that lead can be the factor producing these types of childhood disorders, I'm left with the questions: Why aren't children with such disorders being screened for lead and other metals? Why, if professionals know that lead is a potential cause, aren't they doing anything about it? Why are we continuing to let heavy metals destroy our children's health, intelligence, and future? How many more hundreds of thousands of children have to be subjected to intellectual insult and impairment or become severely mentally retarded before anybody is going to bypass all of the bureaucratic crap and look at this issue seriously?

As several of the studies clearly point out, accurate testing for body burden of lead and metals is of utmost importance. And, when properly diagnosed, assessed, and treated, children's mental/intellectual functioning and motor skills, not to mention their general and long-term health, can improve.

The Centers for Disease Control has published information regarding lead toxicity. Anyone can receive this material by calling the National Lead Information Centre toll-free at 1-800-FYI-LEAD. The CDC information states in no uncertain terms that childhood lead poisoning is one of the most common pediatric health problems in the United States today. The CDC maintains that enough is known about the sources and pathways of lead exposure to make lead poisoning entirely preventable (see the information on sources and prevention in Chapters 9 and 10), and increased efforts could permanently eradicate this disease. It also states that most cases go undiagnosed and untreated. Since virtually all children are at risk for lead poisoning, the CDC recommends that a phase of universal screening should be implemented. Unfortunately, the CDC does not mention the dangers of other metals. As you may have noticed, most of the research has been done on lead; the effects of other metals are only now being studied.

For years lead poisoning was seen as a disease prevalent among residents of the inner city or of industrial towns. Newer research indicates that it is a common childhood health hazard for any group of children — no class, geographical area, race, or ethnic group is spared. In the United States, a recent study found that children in what was believed to be the lowest-risk group — those living outside of central cities — had high levels of lead in their blood.

This problem is not unique to the United States. All industrialized countries pay this heavy toll for their affluence. The U.S. should be commended for acknowledging the problem. I can tell you from experience that it is not a politically or financially easy problem for a government to acknowledge, but facing the problem — the harmful effects of environmental lead — is the first step towards dealing with the issue. Dr. J. Routt Reigart, chairman of the American Academy of Pediatrics environmental health committee and director of general pediatrics at the Medical University of South Carolina in Charleston, recommends that pediatricians pay attention to the CDC statement on lead poisoning which defines high- and low-risk children. He agrees that screening is imperative.

Dr. John F. Rosen — a pediatrician and adviser to the Committee of Childhood Lead Poisoning Prevention in New York City — has said that lead poisoning is the most common preventable disease in young people. He further states that he considers it a national disgrace that such a condition continues to threaten his country's most important resource for the future, its children. He agrees with public health experts who argue that high rates of learning disabilities, school dropouts, and behavior problems are directly related to lead toxicity. Rosen predicts that by the year 2000, the number of children with IQs less than 80 will increase by 50 percent while those with IQs above 120 will decrease by 50 percent, all due to lead poisoning.

High levels of lead have been associated with antisocial behavior, and the serum levels of lead in youths living in inner cities where crime is rampant are much higher than the levels for youths living in rural areas. Could something be done about America's inner city crime by addressing the issue of lead toxicity and, taking it one step further, nutritional status?

The Alliance to End Childhood Lead Poisoning, an advocacy group in Washington, D.C., reported that lead-poisoned children were six times more likely to have reading difficulties. They failed grades at seven times the average rate. In 1992, the *New England Journal of Medicine* published a study conducted by Peter A. Baghurst, Anthony J. McMichael, *et al.*, entitled "Environmental Exposure to Lead and Children's Intelligence at the Age of Seven Years." Their studies in the lead smelter town of Port Pirie, Australia, found developmental problems had already been reported in children by two to four years of age. Re-evaluation of these same children at age seven concluded that there was a strong relationship between a reduction in IQ and elevated antenatal (pregnancy) and postnatal (infancy) blood lead concentrations.

There are many documented cases of chronic lead exposure in children. These cases are usually identified in small communities where extremely high numbers of children have displayed the effects of chronic toxicity. For example, in El Paso, Texas, in 1973, 2700 people living within a four-mile radius of a lead smelter were found to have an excess of lead in their blood. Out of the 2700 people tested with increased lead levels, 131 were children who exhibited signs of neurological damage including nervous system dysfunction, visual impairment, and poor perceptual skills.

Between 1968 and 1970 in Soho County, California, approximately 40 horses and 80 sheep died from lead poisoning. By determining the type of lead compound at an autopsy, testing revealed that 50 percent of the lead came from a lead smelter 30 miles away. The other 50 percent came from auto exhaust emissions. How many people were and are untested and undiagnosed in that county?

There are similar cases in Canada. You can appreciate, of course, that governments and owners of hazardously contaminated property do not wish to advertise these facts. There was a case in Richmond, British Columbia, where animals grazing near an industrial source of lead died from acute lead poisoning. For a few weeks government agents swarmed about dressed in their decontamination suits, test-

ing soil in a neighboring pasture, before advising the proprietor that his land was so contaminated that it could not
sustain domestic animal life. What about human life? Nothing of the event appeared in any of the local papers. There
was no public notice. The proprietor died several years later
from hypertension and heart disease. A residential subdivision has just been built on his land. Welcome, children!

Why aren't we doing anything about this? Environmental
studies have established that lead exposure is commonplace
in this day and age. Lead is not easily contained or removed,
so we have little choice but to look at dealing with this environmental hazard and its degenerating effects upon human life. More importantly, we must start to control its
effects on both children and adults. In the next chapter
Zigurts and I will explain what those effects are, what happens when a human is exposed to unhealthy doses of metals,
and then we'll go on to discuss what can be done to reverse
and prevent metal poisoning.

5

Why are Metals Toxic?

Metals are taken into the body in several different ways. They can be inhaled, eaten, and even absorbed through the skin. After metal particles are inhaled into the lung or ingested into the gut, a portion is slowly absorbed into the bloodstream. Some remains in the lung tissues and some is excreted from the body in the urine and the feces. What is not excreted is eventually deposited in cells of organs and soft tissues of the body. About 90 percent of absorbed lead will end up tightly bound in the skeletal system. If the amount of metal absorbed and sequestered in bones and organs is high enough, noticeable adverse effects will result.

Lead and other metals do not break down in either the environment or in the body. They do not degrade into harmless components, but remain active for long periods of time, and they never go completely away. When lead or cadmium is inhaled, for example, some of the minute particles become trapped in lung tissue. Scientists have observed that there is reduced production of macrophages (cells that remove foreign debris from body tissues) after excessive amounts of lead and cadmium enter the lungs, and this causes a significantly increased risk of respiratory difficulties and infections. After the lead and/or cadmium is removed, some permanent damage is evident in the lungs. It is suspected that both lead and cadmium play a role in some cases of bronchitis and asthma.

The half-life of lead that enters the bloodstream from the

lungs or gut is four to six weeks. This means that the amount of lead absorbed into the bloodstream on any given day will be reduced by half within four to six weeks. Other metals have half-lives of similar length. During this four-to-six-week period, some metal particles will be excreted by the kidneys into the urine and some will pass through the liver which discharges its secretions into the gut. What isn't excreted will be absorbed into bones and body tissues where it will become, in most cases, permanently stored. The half-life of lead and most other heavy metals in body tissues is measured in years — ten to twenty — due to the fact that heavy metals are bound and held strongly in these tissues.

This relatively rapid absorption/excretion means that blood levels reflect only recent exposure. Children or adults experiencing low but constant levels of exposure to metals will have far more of these metals in their bones and soft tissues than in their blood.

Later in life, metals stored in the bones will be released into the bloodstream during demineralization of the bones. This occurs during pregnancy and lactation, when the body is pulling minerals out of the bones to accommodate the fetus's/baby's needs. Any metals present in the bones will be released along with other minerals, and absorbed into the fetal tissues either when the metal passes through the placenta or, later on, through milk while the baby is breastfeeding. A baby can be metal poisoned by its mother! It has been shown that the cognitive functioning of children born to women who have been exposed to high levels of lead is impaired. When we start to think about the numbers of women involved and the risk, it makes sense to encourage women of reproductive age to get tested, especially if they are planning to become pregnant.

Metals will also be released in old age when osteoporosis sets in and bones begin to demineralize. This can cause extreme agitation and mental insufficiency or dementia in the aging adult.

When metals are absorbed out of the bloodstream and stored away in bones, organs, and other tissues, they are still causing damage to every physiological system, but particularly the blood, the kidneys and the nervous system. For example, the presence of lead affects the formation of hemoglobin — the molecule that transports oxygen through the bloodstream to organs and tissues. The resulting anemia or decreased oxygen-carrying capacity of the blood can damage all tissues.

Sensory and motor functions of the central nervous system are affected, causing symptoms ranging from slight changes in memory to overt confusion, hallucinations, dementia, convulsions, coma and even death. Bizarre behavioral changes can occur such as "pica" (the licking, chewing or eating of non-food substances such as dirt, painted wood surfaces and objects, toys, and more unusual items such as match heads). Vision and hearing can be compromised. When cadmium and lead accumulate in the kidneys they block the activation of vitamin D. Without vitamin D, less calcium is absorbed from the digestive tract. As a result, calcium is drawn from bones in order to maintain proper blood calcium levels. This interferes with bone growth and metabolism. Lead and cadmium in the kidneys can also block the elimination of uric acid, a byproduct of protein metabolism. An increase in blood uric acid levels can lead to gout and joint pains. High levels of lead can affect the joints directly, causing symptoms of arthritis; the same effect is caused by high levels of iron in a condition known as hemochromatosis. A person with lead toxicity may develop muscle aches and pains or weakness and atrophy due either to neurological damage or to a direct effect on muscle metabolism. The digestive system may be disturbed producing pain, diarrhea, vomiting, constipation and a loss of appetite. Heavy metals can damage the cardiovascular system, producing chest pain, palpitations, and a rise in blood pressure. This may be due to an acceleration of atherosclerosis (hardening of the arteries) or due to direct damage to the heart muscle itself. Reproductive capacity may be affected both by infertility and impotence. The immune system may be compromised, resulting in fevers, chills and sweats.

Perhaps heavy metal toxicity is seldom diagnosed because it appears as such a wide range of symptoms, and most of these symptoms are attributed to other diseases. Too often we treat the symptoms rather than getting to the bottom of the cause. When a patient has symptoms of arthritis, he is given an anti-inflammatory medication. When a child has fever, he is first given acetaminophen and, if that doesn't work, an antibiotic. If no specific cause for colicky abdominal pain is identified, it is usually treated with pain relievers. Behavioral problems are treated with behavioral modification programs or by various medications. Hallucinations may be treated by anti-psychotics and seizures are treated by anti-convulsants. But all these symptoms could be the result of heavy metal toxicity, and none of the treatments mentioned in this paragraph is going to deal with this cause.

How do metals cause damage?

As I learned about metal toxicity, I was amazed at the varied effects metals can cause and wondered how they could be the culprit in so many different cases. To understand, we have to go back to our high school biology lessons about cells and the body's enzymatic proteins, because metals alter these basic structures of body systems.

The basic unit of all living things, including human beings, is the cell. The components of a cell are the cytoplasm, a cell membrane surrounding the cytoplasm, a variety of structures (for example mitochondria and ribosomes) in the cytoplasm, and a central nucleus contained within a nuclear membrane.

The cell membrane contains complex proteins which transport various components required for cellular metabolism into the cell. These proteins also carry products of cellular metabolism out of the cell. The cell nucleus contains (among other things) the genetic material containing the code which enables the cell to produce various structural and enzymatic proteins.

Enzymatic proteins are a critical factor in metabolism. They act as catalysts or helpers in all chemical reactions. Using vitamins and trace minerals as co-factors, enzymes enable the cell to use carbohydrates, fats, and amino acids to build tissue for structure and to create energy for function. Some enzymes function as repair enzymes, fixing various structures such as the cell membrane, which is in a perpetual state of damage and repair.

To be healthy, a cell requires that all systems within the boundaries of its membrane function properly. Individual cells are then organized into tissues that are specialized to perform precise functions or contribute to a particular structure. These tissues are further organized into organs that carry out certain tasks, *i.e.*, the heart pumps blood, the lungs exchange carbon dioxide and oxygen. All work together to keep the body going, so when the structure or function of any one part is altered or injured, the whole body can suffer.

This is where heavy metals come in. As mentioned, enzymes bind with trace minerals and vitamins to carry out their necessary chemical reactions. Unfortunately, heavy metals such as lead often have a greater affinity for protein enzymes than the necessary trace minerals do. Large quantities of lead, mercury, cadmium, etc. in the body poison essential enzymes by "bumping off" the minerals so the enzymes cannot be properly activated to do their job. For example, if enzymes that repair DNA are poisoned by heavy metals, there is an increased risk that genetic material will be damaged, resulting in an increased rate of tumor growth and birth defects. Heavy metals can interfere with enzymes that repair cell membranes and participate in functions related to the immune system, energy production and storage, and various aspects of detoxification (for example, the removal of poisons carried out by the liver).

Metals also affect the enzymes that deal with "free radicals." (No, we are not talking about escaped political activists or chelation therapists!) Free radicals, otherwise known as reactive oxygen toxic species (ROTS), are atoms or molecules which are "electron hungry" and on the lookout to steal electrons from other atoms or molecules. If a free radical steals an electron from a chemical structure — like a cell membrane — it can damage the integrity of the chemical bonds holding together that structure.

Cells contain enzymes which neutralize these free radicals and protect the integrity of the cell. For example, the superoxide free radical can be neutralized by an enzyme called superoxide dismutase. This enzyme converts superoxide into hydrogen peroxide and molecular oxygen. Because hydrogen peroxide is also damaging, it is further reduced by the catalase enzyme. The catalase and dismutase enzymes require trace minerals like zinc, manganese, and selenium to carry out this neutralization, and vitamin E is a co-factor in the catalase reaction. If zinc and manganese are not able to activate superoxide dismutase to neutralize superoxide free radicals, damage to the cell can occur.

Eventually, as enzymes become clogged with metals, the cells themselves malfunction. This in turn compromises the particular organ or tissue they are a part of. When many cells of organs or body systems become damaged, organ dysfunction becomes evident. For example, if brain cells are damaged, the nervous system stops working properly. As damage to organs increases, the patient gets sicker and sicker.

The point to remember is that lead and other metals may not be the primary cause of health problems, but the presence of toxic metals can undermine the body's normal functioning which will leave a person susceptible to illness, interfere with recovery from a disease, or, in the case of children, hinder development.

Metal toxicity in children vs. adults

While both adults and children are at risk from excessive exposure to lead and other metals, children are much more susceptible to severe damage for several reasons. First of all, a child absorbs toxic metals much more efficiently than does an adult — a child's absorption of lead from the gut is five times as efficient as an adult's. Because of the rapid growth rate and high metabolism of developing children, their little bodies are absorbing larger quantities of nutrients and minerals. Unfortunately, they are also absorbing everything else that is presented to them — including lead and other heavy metals. These metals are taken into the body and absorbed as if they were nutritional. Think of a child weighing eight pounds at birth and by the age of four increasing to a size of thirty to forty pounds. This represents at least a tripling of body mass.

Nutrient requirements are greatest for the most rapidly growing tissues and, in the case of developing children, brain growth is extremely rapid and nearly complete by age six. This means that much of the metal ingested goes into the brain tissue. In general, children are more susceptible to metal toxicity because of their high metabolism relative to their body mass. They consume more of everything per pound of body weight than do adults, they breathe more air and consume more water for their relative body size. (Both air and water are known sources of heavy metal toxicity.) They also excrete less lead and other metals than an adult.

Children also behave in certain ways that make them more susceptible. For instance, children are always putting their fingers in their mouths. They spend more time at ground zero. As toxic metals are frequently found in dust and dirt, on floors and windowsills, children are much more likely to pick up metals such as lead from contaminated windowsills and dusty floors, especially when parents have done renovations to older homes. There have been cases where the renovation of just one room resulted in a child becoming acutely lead poisoned.

An important contributing factor is the child's general health. Children with better nutrition, with higher intakes of trace minerals such as calcium, zinc, magnesium, and, to some degree, iron, tend to be less susceptible than children who are deficient in these trace minerals. Children with inadequate protein intake are also more vulnerable.

As already mentioned, a child may be poisoned long before birth as metals are drawn out of the mother's bones and body tissues, and transferred from the placenta to the fetus along with essential nutrients. The placenta secretes metallothionein, a protein which binds with cadmium and some other heavy metals to prevent their transfer across the placental barrier. If the metallothionein becomes saturated, however, cadmium will pass over to the fetus. Other metals, particularly lead, transfer readily from the mother to the fetus. Researchers have established that umbilical cord blood samples which show that lead levels higher than 7 µg/dl can indicate future learning problems.

Metal exposure continues after birth when the child is breastfeeding. If the mother is exposed to metals in her environment at this time, the metals will end up in her milk. And she will continue to draw stored metals from her body tissues. It is estimated that 500,000 women of childbearing age in North America are lead toxic, having blood lead levels of 10 µg/dl or higher.

Metal poisoning plagues the developing child, accounting for spontaneous abortions, low birth weight, failure to thrive, growth retardation, and delay in cognitive development.

Recent studies from the University of Nebraska Medical Center in Omaha indicate that high levels of lead inhibit the pituitary gland secretion of thyroid-stimulating hormone (TSH). This hormone helps regulate the growth of a child.

The study suggests that excess lead in brain tissue can cause chemical events that will ultimately hinder bone growth and reduce growth in general. This same study reported that children experienced a sudden growth spurt after chelation therapy for lead. This growth spurt was evident in all three of my children after chelation.

Both children and adults can suffer from acute or chronic toxicity. Acute toxicity is the result of excessive exposure to heavy metals in a short period of time. Early symptoms of acute toxicity can include any or all of the following: insomnia, loss of appetite, gastro-intestinal colic, prolonged diarrhea, and unexplained vomiting. In the past, these symptoms were referred to as "painter's colic"; it was a common occurrence for painters to be poisoned by the high lead content in paints.

Symptoms of prolonged excessive exposure to metals are anemia, headaches, and abdominal pain. If exposure is suddenly removed, these symptoms usually stop. If exposure continues, symptoms such as irritability, slow developmental progress, hearing loss, and a dispositional change (usually interpreted as a behavior problem in children) can develop. If excessive exposure is not eliminated and continues for long periods of time — months or years — toxic psychosis with hallucinations, delusions and excitement, delirium, and death can occur.

Chronic toxicity occurs when a person, particularly a child, has had low-level exposure to lead and/or other metals over a long period of time. The most common symptoms of chronic metal poisoning are nervous system dysfunctions affecting cognitive functioning, motor skills, behavior, language skills, etc., and blood cell formation problems like anemia.

It is crucial to understand that in children with obvious behavior and/or learning disabilities, we are not concerned with recent exposure to metals. If the behavior/learning traits have already become obvious, then we should be looking for chronic exposure or the long-term body burden. The metals have already accumulated in the brain and other organs. And, I have to warn you, this is where many doctors need a little educating. That I can tell you from personal experience.

As metal poisoning is not commonly looked for in a young child, a metal-toxic child often becomes misdiagnosed. He or she may end up with labels of attention deficit disorder with or without hyperactivity, pervasive developmental disorder, autistic tendencies, behavior problems, etc. Many of the symptoms of recent exposure to metals are similar to other early childhood illnesses like colic, nausea, loss of appetite, vomiting, diarrhea, etc., and consequently, the metal-toxic child is overlooked and ends up with the chronic form of toxicity. A test for metal poisoning must be part of the doctor's initial diagnosis — in the next chapter we look at methods of testing.

6

Testing for Metal Toxicity

It should be clear by now that before a child is diagnosed with severe behavior problems or learning disabilities, he or she should be tested for body burden of lead and other heavy metals. Keep in mind, too, that early metal exposure produces flu-like symptoms. An infant who suffers prolonged or chronic bouts of colic, nausea, vomiting, irritability, diarrhea, and/or loss of appetite which seem to be occurring for no specific reason should be tested for recent lead and other metal exposure.

A young child living in an area in which there is a high risk of excessive heavy metal exposure (particularly lead, cadmium, or mercury), should also be tested regularly. The United States Environmental Protection Agency (EPA) recommends testing children at six months of age in such cases. It also recommends that every child should be tested at least by one year of age and then every couple of years after that.

A random blood test for lead may be adequate for this purpose but if it is negative, it does not rule out chronic toxicity and it does not rule out the presence of other heavy metals. It is important to note that the presence of other metals can show up in a blood test, but the physician must specifically order the lab to screen for these metals. All metals have a relatively short half-life in the bloodstream, so they are easy to miss and the significance of their presence in a blood sample is difficult to interpret with any degree of accuracy. If they are present in large quantities it could indicate acute toxicity — but, as with lead, an absence in a blood test does not rule out chronic toxicity. Other metals can be more severely toxic than lead or they can combine with relatively small amounts of lead to have a synergistic (multiplying) effect that causes severe neurological compromise. Diagnosis of heavy metal toxicity is the subject of debate and confusion. Mainstream medicine dictates that blood lead levels are the accepted measure, but the level of blood lead indicating toxicity has changed considerably since 1971 — from 60 µg/dl to 10 µg/dl in 1991. Adults appear able to tolerate higher levels of lead without showing signs of toxicity. Children show signs at very low levels and may be acutely affected when their blood lead levels are well below 10 µg/dl. Placental blood levels of 7 µg/dl have been associated with subsequent decrease in academic performance as children mature, and measures below 10 µg/dl have accompanied compromised intellectual development and decreases in IQ , hearing, and growth.

Another debate raging around the usefulness of these readings centers on lead's relatively short half-life in the bloodstream. Blood is a reliable indicator of acute toxicity but not of chronic exposure or total body burden. If there has been recent exposure within two to four weeks resulting in a blood lead level of 10 µg/dl, it is unlikely that a child will display any symptoms of acute or chronic toxicity. These symptoms appear at levels of 40 µg/dl or higher. On the other hand, if exposure has occurred in the past resulting in a steady level of 9 µg/dl, one might expect to find impaired intellectual functioning. For example, one could find blood lead levels below the danger zone in a four-year-old child who may have suffered significant brain damage in the first two years of development due to a constant but low level of lead exposure. The lead will have accumulated in tissues such as bone, brain, and to a lesser extent, the kidneys rather than remaining in the blood. A blood test would not result in a diagnosis of lead poisoning for this child.

So remember this — a random blood test will not represent the concentration of metals in body organs. You can be pretty well guaranteed that a random blood sample from a chronically toxic child will show negative results unless the child has had excessive exposure to lead within the last few weeks.

If you want an accurate measure of the lead and metal burden in the brain and other body tissues, how would you get it? One of the best assessment techniques for measuring body burden of lead is x-ray fluorescence. This testing method uses x-rays which produce one-twentieth the radiation that a dental x-ray produces, yet provide a relatively accurate measure of lead content in bone. Computer software has not been developed yet to measure other heavy metals, but the technology to do so at some future time is available. At the time of the writing of this book, however, x-ray fluorescence is only available in one diagnostic center, in the United States.

Probably the most unintrusive yet significant testing method is an inexpensive, underrated laboratory test called hair elemental analysis. We call it underrated because many physicians do not realize the accuracy of this screening procedure. Over the last twenty years, hundreds of researchers have studied the usefulness of hair samples for providing a profile of the metals and other substances that have been excreted over a period of time equivalent to the age of the hair on an individual's head. The lead that is incorporated into the hair sample reflects the amount of lead that was available in the blood during the time that hair grew.

Although hair elemental analysis is not recommended as a diagnostic tool on its own, many researchers have documented that the elements found in hair samples do relate to nutritional intake, environmental exposure, and to internal biochemical and metabolic conditions. Research has revealed that concentrations of heavy metals in hair provide an accurate and relatively permanent record of exposure.

There is a strong correlation between the concentration of heavy metals in hair and that found in the internal organs. Hair and other organs contain heavy metals at approximately ten times the concentration found in blood. Hair elemental analysis is an important test for evaluating the overall body pool of toxic metals and an indicator of the potential health hazards resulting from synergistic combinations of metals.

Hair analysis is the method of choice for detecting cadmium in the human body. The presence of hair cadmium has been found to relate to brain deterioration, which generally appears as poor concentration, and it has been recognized as being significantly higher in many studies of mildly retarded and learning-disabled children. Dyslexic children in one study had approximately 25 times the hair cadmium as controls.

The EPA cites that hair elemental analysis provides an acceptable measure of an individual's mercury, chromium, and arsenic levels. The EPA further states that hair analysis is at least as accurate as blood and urine sampling for detecting body burden of these metals.

Hair analysis does not provide an accurate body burden evaluation for iron. As a general rule in the interpretation of hair iron analysis, when the level of iron falls outside two standard deviations, high or low, additional methods of testing for more accurate detection of body iron stores should be considered. Medical interventions based solely on the interpretation of hair iron analysis are not recommended.

The EPA also confirms that hair copper levels reflect the body burden of copper. Although hair copper can be distorted by external contamination (for example, hair can be affected when people swim in pools containing copper salts as algae treatment agents), it has been reported to correlate with liver copper levels at a 99.9 percent confidence rate. High hair copper levels may indicate copper toxicity.

The problem with hair, as suggested in the previous paragraph, is that lead and other metals can enter the inactive keratinous structure of hair during its exposure to dirt, dust, sweat, sebum, and other environmental sources (including shampoos, dyes, and other darkening agents, like Grecian Formula, that are applied to the hair). High levels of lead in shower water can contaminate the samples. Hair nickel can be elevated by external exposure to permanents, dyes, and bleaches.

Hair sampled closest to the scalp will provide a more accurate measure of body burden than hair samples taken further out on the shaft. It appears that, as the hair shaft starts to break down, some of the heavy metal content may be lost or washed out. Samples must therefore be new growth, close to the scalp, with the longer ends cut off and discarded. The first inch of hair growth from the scalp is necessary for accurate analysis of current metal burden. Hair must be cut with non-leaded scissors and contained in a paper envelope, plastic bag, or other non-leaded package. If any chemical hair products have been used (permanents, dyes, bleaches, etc.), it is important to document those facts for the laboratory prior to testing so they can be taken into account during the evaluation and interpretation of the samples. (To access immediate hair elemental analysis, see order form at the end of this publication.)

Studies have been done evaluating other tissues. Baby teeth would appear to be good indicators of chronic lead exposure, and one study that I'm aware of did suggest that teeth might be a good indicator of body burden of lead. However, lead is only incorporated into teeth during their rapid growth period; following that, no more lead enters the tooth. Tooth lead therefore reflects the average available lead during the time of growth only, but not before or after.

The most commonly used technique for testing body stores of toxic metals, and a particularly useful one for establishing that they are being excreted from the body, is "provocative urine testing." In this method, a urine sample is taken before and after a chelating agent is given to a child. The chelator may be in the form of an oral chelating agent, such as Cuprimine, or it may be an intravenous chelating agent such as ethylene diamine tetracetic acid — EDTA. The chelator is the "provocative" part of the test because it challenges or "provokes" the metal ions and pulls them out of the body tissues. Metals are either in solution in the human body (which is composed of 57 percent water) or they are bound to various tissues and chemicals. The chelator has a stronger attraction for metal particles than does water or most body tissues, so the particles are taken up by the chelating agent and are eventually excreted. The process of elimination depends upon the chelator being used. Some are eliminated intact or unprocessed through the kidney, others through the liver and bowels. Some are excreted by both routes and may even leave the body through perspiration.

Following one or two days of treatment with an oral chelating agent, or a single dose of an intravenous chelating agent, a chelated urine sample is collected. Results from this sample are compared to pre-treatment measurements. A chelated urine sample that shows excessive metals being excreted is an indication that metals are being sequestered in the body tissues. There shouldn't be metals present in the urine that is being tested. Heavy metals do not belong in the human body at any level. Excessive excretion of heavy metals suggest that the child (or adult) is metal toxic. The results of provocative urine tests appear to parallel results found by x-ray fluorescence and hair sampling. The physician must be sure to screen for all toxic metals. Finding a low lead level does not exclude the possibility of heavy metal poisoning caused by either a combination of lead and another metal or another metal by itself.

There are two main methods of chelation testing, the 8- or 24-hour urine collection and the urine stress test. The former is a simple test in which all urine excreted from the body is collected for a designated period of time after the administration of a chelator. As the medication must first be absorbed, and then pass into body tissues and cross the blood-brain barrier before it starts pulling out metal ions, the urine is collected several hours after ingestion of the chelator. In our testing, we began the chelator on day one. After the first morning urine was flushed the second day, the subsequent samples were collected, including the first urination of the third morning. This method of testing provides a full 24-hour evaluation of the heavy metals excreted from the body.

The "before and after" urine stress test is another simple, yet effective method to measure tissue accumulation of metals. One random urine sample (without provocation by chelating agents) should be obtained for elemental analysis. This will indicate the amount of metals expelled by the body on a daily basis and reveals typical, recent exposure. The next sample should be taken on the second day after commencement of an oral chelating agent. The first morning urine should be discarded. The second, two hours after the morning chelating agent has been administered, should be collected and analysed for elements.

Once you have samples of hair or urine, you have to find the right laboratory. At present, most hospital laboratories in Canada and the United States do not test hair or urine samples for metal excretion patterns. Private local laboratories sometimes do, but their fees are usually not covered by medical insurance. Our experience in Canada is that private labs are seldom requested to do such testing on human tissues or fluids, and their fees are generally quite high. The U.S. appears to be further ahead in this regard, reflecting more widespread acknowledgement of the health hazards of heavy metals and the importance of metal screening.

Quality control and cost are two important issues. When hair analysis first became available there was an abundance of opportunists competing for a fad-driven market. Results were inconsistent and hair analysis fell into disrepute. Over the years, however, better equipment and techniques, along with a weeding out of fly-by-night labs, have resulted in government-accredited labs that can pass quality control inspections. There are several labs in the United States which we favor because of their experience, quality of service, excellent reporting, and lower cost. Accuracy and consistency, as you can understand, are the two main criteria. For any of these tests that we have described, expect to pay anywhere from US$25 to US$60 depending on the type of tissue sample and which lab you use.

Two laboratories in the U.S. which have provided excellent elemental analysis of both urine and hair samples for many of the children described in this book are:

Doctor's Data Incorporated
c/o Doctor's Data Inc.
PO Box 111, 30W101 Roosevelt Road
West Chicago, IL 60185
1-800-323-2784

Omegatech
King James Medical Laboratory
24700 Center Ridge Road, Suite 113
Cleveland, OH 44145
1-800-437-1404

In a case where the results are equivocal, a decision about commencing chelation treatment has to be made based on the risk of medication or treatment versus the benefit. Fortunately, most chelating agents are safe to use in the hands of a conscientious physician.

Before any of these agents are administered, a physician must start with a thorough history focusing on sources of heavy metal exposure, the route of intake, and which systems are primarily affected. Hair analysis can be useful in this instance and could precede a provocative urine test. The physician must take sensitivities and allergies into account.

A physical examination needs to be done with the necessary lab tests: white and red blood cell counts, platelet count, liver and kidney function tests. In some cases it is necessary to do an electrocardiograph, thyroid function tests, sugar levels, and blood tests measuring levels of sodium, potassium, calcium, and magnesium. Blood iron levels should be monitored. A patient with a history of anemia and metal poisoning should be tested for red and white blood cell levels before, during, and after a course of treatment.

It is also important to monitor trace mineral status as minerals may need to be supplemented, either because they have been displaced by the presence of heavy metals or because they can also be pulled out of the body by chelators. While a patient is undergoing treatment, oral supplementation with trace minerals, antioxidant vitamins, a diet consisting of lots of fiber, large amounts of water, and increased physical activity are necessary.

During prolonged treatment, the patient's chemical tests need to be assessed on a regular basis. Changes in symptoms and behavior must be monitored. Patients should inform their physician of any rapid change in their symptoms.

More thorough guidelines for diagnosis and treatment of heavy metal toxicities using chelation agents can be obtained by mailing in the form at the end of the book.

Understanding chelation

So what exactly is going on when a metal-toxic child or adult is given chelation therapy? The word "chelation" is derived from the Greek word "chele," or "claw" of a crab. It describes the way metal ions are grasped by a chelating agent to form a stable metal-chelate complex which can then be removed. The historical foundation of chelation dates back to 1893 when Alfred Werner founded the concept of coordination chemistry. Prior to that, the only chemical bond that was understood was that in which, simply speaking, a positively charged atom was attracted to and combined with a negatively charged atom or particle. The theory of coordination chemistry involved the complexing of a positively charged atom within a molecule consisting of complex ring structures of orbiting electrons. The atom was strongly bound to the molecule as they shared several electrons.

One of the earliest industrial applications of chelation occurred in the early 1900s when the textile and printing industries used citric acid to remove calcium from hard water because the calcium tended to stain various dyes. In the 1930s, the Nazi government in Germany wanted to reduce the import of citric acid from abroad. Frederick Munz noted that there was a similarity between citric acid and a chemical known as nitrile-triacetic acid; on testing this substance he found it to be an effective chelator of calcium.

The use of poison gases such as the arsenic-based Lewisite as weapons of war prompted scientists to develop an antidote for arsenic poisoning. Their research led to the synthesis of BAL or British Anti-Lewisite in 1945. Subsequent research led to the development of ethylene diamine tetracetic acid (EDTA) and other chelating compounds.

Also in the 1940s, Dr. Frederick Bersworth filed a patent application in the United States for the commercial production of EDTA through another chemical process. With Bersworth's support, Martin Rubin, a chemist at Georgetown University, investigated biological uses for EDTA, focusing on calcium metabolism. This research resulted in the use of EDTA as an anticoagulant for the storage of blood and blood products. EDTA is still used for this purpose today.

Its first use in human beings was in 1947, also at Georgetown University. Dr. Charles Geschickter, a colleague of Martin Rubin, administered an EDTA-nickel complex to a dying breast cancer patient as a form of chemotherapy. No therapeutic benefit was found, but no toxic effects were observed either. Further studies that used EDTA to dissolve kidney and bladder stones also demonstrated that it was a relatively safe drug.

In 1951 the first reports of the use of EDTA for lead poisoning were published by Dr. Norman Clarke. He subsequently published a paper on the use of EDTA for atherosclerosis. Many of the patients he was treating for lead poisoning saw their symptoms of cardiovascular disease lessen or disappear when they received EDTA.

The favorable results obtained by detoxifying adults resulted in the use of EDTA for detoxifying lead-poisoned children. It is still the treatment of choice in major centers dealing with childhood lead poisoning. Over the years, EDTA has proven itself useful for the treatment of many conditions where either heavy metal toxicity or increased calcification of tissues is a problem. The recent recognition by the Centers for Disease Control that lead poisoning is a significant epidemiological problem has led to sophisticated programs of identification, diagnosis, treatment and prevention. Research has led to the development of new chelating agents including dimercaptosuccinic acid (DMSA), desferoxamine (Desferal), and D-penicillamine (Cuprimine), and dimercaptopropanesulfonic acid (DMPS). Some amino acids also appear to have chelating properties. These include argenine, glycine, lysine, and cystine.

Because EDTA is poorly absorbed through the gut, it requires intravenous administration. The recent development of several oral chelating agents which are reasonably well absorbed through the gut have given the chelating physician a broader choice of medications. This has been particularly useful for children who are often too agitated or frightened to sit still for the time required to administer intravenous medication, from ten or fifteen minutes for DMPS, to three hours or more for EDTA.

If a person has allergies to any of the chelating agents, the physician now can choose another chelator. For instance, Cuprimine is a penicillin derivative. Patients with known penicillin hypersensitivity can avoid the use of this agent.

DMSA contains sulphur, so a patient with a sulphur sensitivity can be given an alternative. With more experience we are learning that some chelating agents are more effective than others in treating certain types of heavy metal toxicity. For instance, the best chelator for iron overload is Desferal. Mercury is chelated by both DMSA and DMPS. However, caution must be exercised in this area. There have been cases of convulsions and severe constipation with abdominal colic when DMSA is used for mercury poisoning. It is believed that these symptoms occur because some mercury is reabsorbed as it passes through the liver and bowels. This can cause bowel paralysis or obstruction, and signs of acute toxicity.

Besides allergic reactions or possible reabsorption of metals, a patient needs to be monitored for kidney failure caused by the rapid elimination of heavy metals through the kidneys. Kidney failure in this case is usually reversible, but these side effects mean that excretion of metals should be gradual and must be carefully monitored. Dosages of chelating agents must be carefully prescribed and, at times, may need to be decreased.

Finally, a less clearly understood phenomenon is that certain tissues tend to have a stronger affinity for one metal as opposed to another. For example, the brain tends to have a stronger affinity for aluminum and mercury. Post-mortem studies show little, if any, mercury or aluminum is eliminated from brain tissue over time. The blood-brain barrier may have something to do with that. Therefore, in selecting an appropriate chelating agent, one not only needs to know the chemical binding strength of a specific chelating agent for a specific metal (*i.e.*, if the chelator will be able to pull it out of body tissues) but must also consider, in the case of aluminum or mercury, whether that chelating agent can cross the blood-brain barrier.

Acute toxicity

Up to now we have mostly been talking about testing for chronic metal poisoning, but we would like to say a bit about diagnosing and treating acute metal toxicity. It can cause any or all of the following symptoms: insomnia, loss of appetite, gastro-intestinal colic, prolonged diarrhea, and unexplained vomiting. If the source of exposure to metals is removed, these symptoms will clear up. If not, you can expect anemia, headaches, abdominal pain, irritability, slow developmental progress, hearing loss, and a dispositional change or behavior problems. Severe cases may lead to toxic psychosis with hallucinations, delusions, extreme agitation and excitement, and death.

Acute lead toxicity has long been determined by the measurement of a blood sample. There are some common guidelines that have been set by which to diagnose and treat acute lead toxicity. As we've said again and again, the point at which lead is recognized as a problem has drastically changed over the last few decades as research is beginning to show severe health hazards and associated physical and mental damage occurring at levels previously thought to be safe. Although there is no absolute single level at which acute toxicity begins, there are some common guidelines that have been recommended. One set of guidelines is used to determine both chronic and acute toxicity in children and adults. This is ironic, as children and adults are affected very differently, at different levels of exposure. The currently accepted guidelines, recommended by the Centers for Disease Control in October 1991, are set out in the table on page 79.

As the table shows, the CDC states levels of less than 10 µg/dl do not indicate lead poisoning. At levels exceeding 10 µg/dl, some effort is made to prevent further exposure. These efforts focus on tracking down the source of lead and removing it or covering it up. A full home inspection is not

μg/dl	Class	Recommended action
< 10	I	Not considered to be lead poisoned
10-14	IIA	Prevention, and rescreen more frequently
15-19	IIB	Nutritional/educational interventions, and rescreen more frequently
20-44	III	Possible pharmacological treatment
45-69	IV	Chelation therapy administered
> 69	V	Medical emergency

recommended at levels below 14 μg/dl, although the patient is counselled about how to avoid further exposure. Follow-up blood testing is recommended in three months. No treatment is prescribed to remove lead already in the body.

At levels between 15 and 19 μg/dl a more careful history is obtained. People displaying levels of 15 μg/dl or more receive individual case management including nutritional support and education to reduce the chance of further exposure. More frequent screening is encouraged, and intensive counselling and environmental investigation is done. Remediation (clean-up, cover-up, and/or removal) of the cause is also done, resources permitting.

At levels exceeding 20 μg/dl, further medical assessment is recommended. This does not mean that chelation is provided, but further testing is done to assess the damage that may have already occurred: bloodwork to check for iron deficiency anemia, kidney and liver function; urinalysis to check for kidney damage; and neurological testing for obvious neurological manifestations — i.e., stupor, seizures, gross and/or fine motor incoordination, behavioral changes, etc. Learning disabilities and language development delays are not assessed until levels reach 20 μg/dl or over.

Depending upon the availability of qualified resources, a home inspection may be a part of this process. Additional methods known to be effective in determining body burden, such as hair elemental analysis, provocative urine testing, and x-ray fluorescence, can be employed, but many physicians report that they simply do not know how to begin assessing and treating this problem.

In cases which exceed 20 µg/dl up to 44 µg/dl, chelation treatment may be recommended. This is left up to the treating physician's discretion.

In cases which exceed 45 µg/dl, both medical interventions (chelation therapy) and environmental interventions are deemed to be necessary. Where blood lead levels are above 70 µg/dl, the adult or child is dealt with as a medical emergency and both medical and environmental investigations and remediations must be provided.

The issue of acute metal toxicity is a serious health concern. However, the medical profession is turning a deaf ear to the fact that the effects of chronic toxicity are far more damaging, to the point that some of the damage becomes irreversible. By focusing only on high blood lead levels, doctors are missing chronic toxicity and the associated damage that could be treated. For example, we recently heard about a pediatrician who had tried to introduce hair testing at a local hospital. The hospital refused to allow it, leaving the physician with the option of blood lead testing only. She ordered blood tests for all her autistic and ADD patients, but of course all tests came back below the 10 µg/dl benchmark. Because of this, the whole area of chronic metal toxicity has been missed in these children. Their parents have been left with the assumption that their children are not metal toxic.

So at the risk of sounding repetitive, we'd like to emphasize the following points.

When looking at a blood lead measurement, you will see only a reasonable estimation of exposure over the last four to six weeks. Now, just for a minute, assume that a child's exposure started when he was an infant and continued until approximately age four — the age when blood testing for lead was finally commenced. Wouldn't it be reasonable to assume that this exposure (particularly if it was coming from water, paint dust, or air) was present every single day of that child's life? And if it was, imagine the accumulation of toxic metal in his body tissues. A blood lead measurement may indicate 3 μg/dl, even though the child's body may be saturated with lead and other metals that had been accumulating from what might be a fairly consistent blood level of 3 μg/dl every day over the last four years and prenatally. He may already have neurological damage from this accumulation, which has been rapidly absorbed over a period of intense growth and development, a time known to be one of excessive absorption of all elements, toxic metals included. A blood test cannot measure the body burden of lead in a child. It can be useful to measure recent exposure. It cannot and will not meaningfully apply to chronic exposure.

Lead is only a small part of the spectrum of metals which should be tested for in children displaying the described symptoms. Keep in mind that cadmium, aluminum, mercury, tin, copper, nickel, arsenic, etc. will also cause these symptoms. A blood lead level will not indicate the presence of any other heavy metals known to cause the same types of neurological deterioration. A blood test will miss metals that can interact with lead to cause major problems. Let's not ignore this important piece of information.

By continuing to use a blood lead measurement, officials are ignoring chronically toxic children. Officials are concerned about preventing metal toxicity and they make no bones about it. All of the literature available regarding lead toxicity states that the medical community is actively looking at prevention of lead toxicity in children . . . prevention only. Why? Because they know the damage that lead causes in young children. But why won't they consider treating the thousands, perhaps millions of children who are already displaying the effects of lead and other metals?

We don't have an answer for that question, but we can tell you about some of these toxic children who have been treated and have shown some amazing recoveries.

7

Who Are the Affected Children?

When the Centers for Disease Control reports that one out of six preschoolers have blood lead levels that can cause neurological damage, it is not even beginning to address the other metals and their extremely harmful effects, both on their own and in combinations which have been shown to multiply the actual damage from toxicity. The one-in-six statistic may be a fairly conservative estimate.

So, we ask, who are the affected children? Heavy metal toxicity is not a health hazard limited to certain neighborhoods or socioeconomic groups as was once believed. Metal toxicity knows no boundaries. All children are potentially at risk. The affected children are children from my community, from your community, and likely from every community. The affected children do not just live in the inner city, in run-down housing, or next door to a lead smelter or battery recycling plant. My children, for example, lived in a middle-class neighborhood in a large residential area. Our house was not very old. Our yard was landscaped, fenced, and well kept. We had a lovely park right down the street. My children were well cared for and had all the luxuries that modern-day children could have. We followed the recommended infant food guide for their early nutritional requirements. We were your average, typical family.

After we discovered Cam and Brett were suffering from the effects of metal toxicity, I was more than surprised to find that several of their Playcare peers lived close to us. In fact, several of them were living next door to each other. After studying the effects of toxic metals on children's health, warning bells suddenly began to ring in my mind. How could rare occurrences such as autistic tendencies, attention deficit disorder, hyperactivity, language delay, and gross behavioral and emotional problems be occurring in almost every house on a block, when the actual estimated occurrence of these disorders is fairly rare? Wasn't this a little bit unusual? Certainly it required some investigating.

Richmond Drive (all names and addresses have been changed) is in an area of North Vancouver which boasts some of the oldest houses in our community. It is located directly off a main roadway which was, incidentally, one of the first major roadways in the city. It is also on the edge of what used to be a mining area. There used to be a small-time copper mine there, I believe, and this same area was a base for shingle mills when the community was originally established. It is one of the first recipients of local water runoff coming straight from the watershed of surrounding mountains.

Bobby Smith was a five-year-old child living on Richmond Drive who had been diagnosed with autistic tendencies. He had an attention deficit and was hyperactive, impulsive, language delayed, and had emotional and behavioral problems. He also had poor fine and gross motor skills. He had been on medications for seizures since he was approximately nine months old. The cause: unknown. Bobby required constant attention and supervision for his own safety. His parents were devastated, living with the assumption that Bobby's disabilities would be permanent, lifelong, and severe.

When I gave Bobby's parents information regarding heavy metals and their effects on young developing children, they were aghast. They lived in a old house which they had renovated during the time that Bobby was conceived. As a baby, Bobby was colicky. He had gut symptoms as an infant (gastric upset, nausea, vomiting, diarrhea, etc.). However, many other children do too, so his parents hadn't been overly concerned.

Bobby had progressed through the early motor milestones at the appropriate ages. Then at approximately nine months old, for no recognizable diagnostic reason, he suddenly had a seizure. Although extensive testing was performed to try to diagnose the underlying cause of the seizure, none was found. He was prescribed anti-convulsant therapy from then on.

Bobby continued to progress normally until about age two when he became increasingly impulsive and hyperactive. His language was delayed, and he seemed to have trouble with verbal comprehension. More extensive testing was done and no underlying cause was found. By age three, Bobby had been through many tests. He was diagnosed with autistic tendencies, and started going to a special needs preschool program which focused on behavior management and language development, with speech therapy also provided. He was generally anxious, agitated, irritable, sometimes aggressive, and had a poor attention span. He was clearly learning disabled and required extensive interventions to keep on task.

Bobby's parents were more than willing to try anything which might improve his situation and, hopefully, his potential. They recognized that their son had been at extreme risk for accidental heavy metal exposure as an infant and were eager to commence testing. His test results indicated an excessive accumulation of lead, copper, cadmium, aluminum, arsenic, and nickel, and a deficiency in lithium and other essential elements. Within the first month following a three-day test with chelating agents, Bobby's anxiety and agitation decreased noticeably. It was not only noticeable to his parents and myself, but also to those caring for him in his preschool setting. In fact, a few months later Mrs. Smith was advised that Bobby didn't qualify for a special needs daycare subsidy any longer because his condition had improved so much that he no longer met the disability criteria for this program.

Bobby's mother was elated when she told her pediatrician of the test results and the accompanying improvements in her child. The pediatrician was furious. He brought his colleague into the room and the two of them lit into her. They told her that, although perhaps her child should be tested for lead, the traditional method of testing was a blood sample. They further told her that she should not be pursuing this avenue of investigation, that it was dangerous and could be harmful to her child, and that until Bobby's anti-convulsant medication was discontinued in another year, she should not be consulting any other physician or following any other types of treatment — especially chelation — without their consent.

They left her feeling frightened, intimidated, and confused. Bobby's condition was improving, after all. When they told her that they would not support this type of medical treatment, she felt she had no choice but to discontinue it. There were other children in the neighborhood undergoing chelation therapy for metal toxicity, so Bobby's mother decided to monitor them and possibly re-establish the treatment once Bobby's anti-convulsants were discontinued.

One of the children she observed was Ben Wong, Bobby's next door neighbor. He was one year younger than Bobby and although he appeared physically normal, he had atypical motor development. He displayed gastro-intestinal irritation as an infant and he liked to eat unusual non-food substances as a toddler. Ben had attentional problems, was hyperactive, impulsive, agitated, irritable, and aggressive. His language was delayed and he had noticeable behavioral and emotional problems.

Bobby's mother shared her information on metal toxicity with Ben's mom, who was curious but waited to see what Bobby's test results were. When the results came in and the improvements were obvious, Ben underwent testing. His test results also indicated an excessive body burden of metal, but when his mother consulted her pediatrician (inciden tally, the same one as Bobby's) she was told not to proceed with the treatment or further investigations. The pediatrician instead ordered a blood sample to be drawn and tested. Although the blood sample did indicate some lead in the bloodstream, the level was not high enough to warrant further investigation under the current guidelines. Other heavy metals were not assessed. To the best of my knowledge, no further testing was done. Ben moved away from the neighborhood.

Four-year-old Brian Muran lived right behind Bobby's house. Mrs. Smith and Ms Muran had often commented on the fact that both of their children, and other neighboring children, displayed the same types of handicaps. Brian was hyperactive, impulsive, irritable, aggressive, agitated, emotionally problematic, had an attention deficit, and displayed some autistic tendencies. He was language delayed and he was going to be attending a segregated preschool for special needs children.

The information was shared with Brian's mom who immediately took her son to be tested for body burden of heavy metals. Brian's tests also indicated excessive body burden of metals. Upon treatment, his condition improved significantly. His agitation and anxiety decreased noticeably and his language skills began to improve.

Harry Singh was a four-year-old boy living across the street from the other three boys. I had met his mother initially through a neighbor of mine and we had further contact as our husbands worked for the same employer. She once described her son's learning and developmental problems, which were similar to those of the other children mentioned. At that point I had no idea that she lived on Richmond Drive and was stunned when I found out. In her search for underlying factors contributing to her son's neurological disabilities, Mrs. Singh had exhausted all of the traditional medical options. She was at her wit's end trying to cope with physicians and behavior therapists concerning her son's mental challenges. When she read about metal toxicity, she immediately saw all the connections: the older home, the renovations, the old water pipes, and the first-draw tap water syndrome. She recognized the same gastrointestinal problems in her child. She had often consulted the doctor for her son's colic, excessive screaming, crying, obvious agitation, and anxieties as an infant. Now it all made complete sense and she was anxious to explore this new avenue of investigation as she was sure that her son was metal toxic. She was absolutely right. After three days of chelation to collect the provocative urine samples, Harry's condition improved noticeably. His anxiety and agitation were significantly reduced. His emotional stability improved. Mrs. Singh already knew what the test results would indicate.

They showed excessive excretion of lead, cadmium, aluminum, arsenic, nickel, and copper. Further treatments and tests indicated the same, and with each successive treatment there were more improvements. Harry's parents were thrilled. Their son was becoming much more manageable. Harry, who had been on the waiting list for a special needs segregated preschool for handicapped children, was now able to attend a regular preschool.

This is not to say that he has completely recovered. Harry still lacks some social skills (mainly a disinterest in seeking out social interactions with other children; he prefers adult stimulation), but he has proven to be a bright, responsive child with more potential than he was ever given credit for. His parents are impressed and describe him as completely different from the child they had before he was treated.

Eight months after these children were evaluated for excessive body burden of heavy metals, another concerned mother called me. Mrs. Godfrey had been looking for me for some months and was eventually given my name by a pharmacist across town. She hadn't known about the children on Richmond Drive, but she had seen an article in our local newspaper about my twin boys and their metal toxicity, and she had recognized similar types of disorders in her two children. She was fairly sure her children had been exposed to heavy metals as young children. I shared some information with her and we continued to chat. When she gave me her address to drop off more literature, I was shocked to hear she lived one street over from Richmond Drive. She said all of the mothers on the block were anxious to have this information because the majority of children living there had neurological disturbances. Eventually we identified five children on that one city block who might be victims of metal toxicity.

The mothers from Richmond Drive told me about several other children who used to live on their street who had displayed obvious neurological problems. One recalled a chilling story of a local toddler who died a few years earlier from a brain tumor.

Just recently I received a phone call from a mother who had moved from Richmond Drive and now lives in Ontario. Both her children have some subtle and not-so-subtle neurological deficits. She had heard through a neighbor of mine that I was helping to establish effective testing for such children, and she wanted her kids tested. Subsequent reports on both children showed cadmium levels that were extremely elevated. I've never seen them quite so high in a child.

My family originally lived fairly close to these children — about eight blocks away from Richmond Drive. I recently ran into my former neighbor's brother-in-law. When I asked him how her children were doing he said that they were having problems. When I asked if they were problems like attentional difficulties, hyperactivity, impulsiveness, learning disabilities, etc. his eyes practically popped out of his head. Those were the problems. In fact, he said, the young boy was having such extreme difficulties that he was now on Ritalin and his mother, a devoted super-mom, could no longer handle him nor care for him. He had been sent to live with his father who was also struggling to manage this unmanageable child.

When I passed metal toxicity information to my former neighbor, she recognized all the same signs and symptoms in her children — the gut problems as toddlers, the incredible anxiety and agitation, the language delay, the attentional problems. She was left with little doubt that her children are also victims of chronic heavy metal toxicity. They are now being tested.

The story of Richmond Drive and surrounding area illustrates two common denominators that surfaced as Zigurts and I began to hear from parents of metal-toxic children. The first thing that became obvious was the clusters of children in our community experiencing gross neurological problems. There were streets full of them. And accompanying parallel streets full of them! There were children living side by side who had gross neurological problems and nobody ever seemed to question this coincidence.

The second obvious fact was that there were, in many cases, multiple occurrences in a single family. Two, three, even four children in one family were all experiencing neurological difficulties. Many of these families were led to believe that their problems were genetic, though none had undergone testing to prove this.

These common denominators led me to look for a cause that might be responsible for such an epidemic of toxicity. Could it be the deteriorating paint from the houses? Could it be the renovations done on some of the houses? Could it be the amount of metals present in the first draw of tap water that's been sitting in lead or copper pipes, or the fact that our water supply, as it becomes more acidic, is leaching more metals from our house plumbing into our drinking water? Is it the soil which has been contaminated by many decades of leaded car emissions? Or is it contamination due to poor standards (or no standards) of control for the disposal of toxic metals common to copper mines (lead, arsenic, cadmium) or shingle mills (arsenic) of the pioneer days? Could it be the poor air quality, polluted by leaded gas emissions that are blown across the city and eventually trapped against our mountainside? These children were breathing that air all through their infancy.

All of these factors could have contributed to the excessive exposure and subsequent accumulation of toxic metals in these children. There are probably more sources of exposure that I don't even know about in our area.

As word about the dramatic improvements in children's conditions after removal of excessive metal burden leaked out, many other parents from our community contacted me. I knew many of them already. When you have children with particular mental handicaps, you end up at all the same schools, meetings, and workshops designed for dealing with special needs children and their multitude of difficulties. Many of these parents were concerned that their children, too, had been exposed to excessive environmental metals during infancy.

One family that sticks out in my mind lived next to a major highway. They lived in an older home which they had renovated during their son's infancy. Although their daughter, aged nine, didn't display any overt signs of metal toxicity, their son David, six years old, certainly did.

I was familiar with David Fredriksen because he had attended Playcare with Cameron and Brett. Although he functioned at a higher level then my twins, David displayed obvious signs of anxiety and severe agitation. His speech was delayed and he had some problems with verbal comprehension. Although he had seen countless specialists during his early years, none had ever suspected metal toxicity, even though he was a severely colicky baby, was constantly crying and upset, and had displayed the gastro-intestinal symptoms associated with metal ingestion. But, again, this seems to be a fairly common pediatric problem.

David reached the physical motor milestones at the appropriate dates, but as a toddler his gross and fine motor skills were clearly not those of a child his age. At five years old he had some language skills and, with the help of speech therapy, was making good progress with communication. He continued to be very anxious and easily upset, though, and changes in routine were almost intolerable for him. He was also hypersensitive to sounds; loud noises left David hiding under a desk or clinging to an adult. Although he had made some progress with his social skills, David was clearly behind other children of his age group, and other children could easily spot his inadequacies.

Although we didn't suspect excessive metals would be discovered in this child (we had only dealt with obviously and grossly affected children up until this point), it turned out David was suffering from metal toxicity. After the first three-day administration of chelating agents, David made sudden, impressive gains in his overall performance. His family was extremely excited, and his mother took the information to her pediatrician, Dr. Craig, who worked in the same office as Bobby Smith's doctor. By now Dr. Craig had heard about many recovering children from our community. Several of them were on his caseload. He took the opportunity to question David's mom. "Let me play the devil's advocate," he suggested to her. "Do you really think that these changes are a result of chelation therapy for removal of heavy metals?"

Ms Fredriksen was firm and confident in her response. She said that, because these changes happened so rapidly and in exact conjunction to the time of treatment for removal of excess heavy metals from her son's body, there was no doubt in her mind that the treatment was the reason for the changes. If they had occurred over a longer period of time, or occurred more subtly, she might have suspected that they were just maturational changes. "But it hasn't been that way," she pointed out. "You know how disabled David was by his condition. Look at him now. And everybody is noticing the changes in him. No, this is not incidental. This is the result of chelation therapy for heavy metal toxicities. There is no doubt in my mind."

After subsequent testing and continued removal of excessive metals from David's body (he had low to moderate concentrations of lead, cadmium, arsenic, copper, and aluminum — the combination adding up to an excessive total concentration of toxins), improvements continued rapidly. Treatment was conducted over the course of the summer months between kindergarten and Grade 1. When David returned to school in September, his kindergarten teacher exclaimed to Ms Fredriksen, "You have a different child now!" She had never seen such rapid and positive change in a young child's behavior and personality.

David's sister was also tested, displayed a similar pattern of metal concentrations in her body, and was treated for their removal. Her parents now find her calmer than before. Her concentration skills have improved. And she was never even thought to be having difficulties.

So here we have some children who live in my own neighborhood. Now I'd like to tell you about a group of children from the other side of the community.

Kelly and Casey O'Connor lived about ten miles away. Kelly, a seven-year-old girl, and Casey, her five-year-old brother, were both struggling with mental handicaps. Kelly's problems were not as extensive as Casey's, but they were serious enough to stamp her with the label "autistic tendencies," and she required special services and supports to help her development and integration into the community and school settings.

Casey was severely affected and showed almost exactly the same behavior and lack of cognitive development and language as my twins. When I first met him he was naked, standing up on the windowsill, making completely incoherent sounds — it struck me that he was an exact replica of my children before removal of excessive metal burden.

To further arouse my suspicions, both children were infants when their house underwent extensive renovations. They were fed water (in formula, juices, foods, etc.) straight from the tap. Mrs. O'Connor described their old car which she transported her babies in, and told of an incident in which her mother had commented on the constant smell of gasoline in the car (leaded gasoline, that is). Mr. O'Connor related an incident which occurred at the time his children were babies. He had just commenced landscaping their home, and had truckload after truckload of soil brought into his yard. The neighbor asked where he bought it from and, on learning the company's name, told Mr. O'Connor that he heard this company was delivering contaminated soil from landfill sites.

Mr. and Mrs. O'Connor, after reading about toxic metals and their effects on young children, were horrified. When they read of all the ways children could be exposed to toxins, they were afraid they had just about done it all. And despite multitudes of medical assessments and consultations with children's specialists and autism specialists over the course of many years, no one had ever suggested metal toxins to be at the root of these children's problems.

In order to investigate metals as a possible cause of their mental handicaps, Kelly and Casey were first seen by their family physician (incidentally, he was also my family physician). He ordered blood tests, which indicated the presence of an "acceptable" level of lead. Other metals were not assessed. However, this physician was aware of the procedure that my twin sons had gone through and agreed that Kelly and Casey should commence further investigation for metal toxins.

Chelation test results showed that Kelly and Casey were carrying enormous concentrations of toxic metals in their body tissues, and after their first treatment everyone involved in working with these two children noted their decreased levels of anxiety and agitation. Casey, a child who, like my twins, had previously been awake five or more times virtually every night since his birth, began to sleep through the entire night. Both children were now noticeably calmer and had an improved ability to focus on, and stay on, task. And this ability to stay on task meant improvements were beginning to occur in many other areas of their cognitive development.

In a letter to me, Mrs. O'Connor wrote that there was no doubt in her mind that her children were victims of chronic metal toxicity. She had pursued genetic testing for Fragile X Syndrome, a genetic mutation responsible for profound mental retardation in families, and found that her children did not possess this mutated gene. With this eliminated as a possible cause of her children's autism, there were only a few other factors that could have produced such an aberration. Environmental toxins were one of them.

Mrs. O'Connor also wrote in the letter about her family's pursuit of testing and treatment for chronic metal exposure, and the improvements that she has witnessed as a result.

> It is obvious that the practice of lead chelation is very unorthodox in the eyes of the Canadian medical profession, and doctors as well as government are in great need of education and empirical evidence before it will become an acceptable method of treatment. Parents as well have a great need for education and resources to enable them to make informed decisions as to treatment for their children without fear of reprisals or intimidation . . .
>
> Although not all problems/symptoms described as autistic have been eliminated [in her children], the improvement in our family quality of life has been phenomenal, and I feel we need to assist other families to pursue chelation therapy. It would be easy to say that most of the above progress would have occurred through natural development and maturity, however

the co-incidences and sudden improvements noted by family and teachers have convinced us of the merits of chelation therapy accompanied by a program of mineral build-up.

Which brings me to Kelly and Casey's neighbor. Right across the street, their two-year-old neighbor was in the process of being labelled with autistic tendencies. Much like all of the other children described in this chapter, Danny Petrenko appeared to be a normal little boy with average development. However, Danny displayed some unusual gut problems. He was a little colicky, spat up, cried a lot, and seemed to be somewhat distressed as an infant. Danny had no language skills, poor eye contact, poor comprehension of language, and did not socialize. He had a sister a couple of years older. Although not so difficult as the baby, she was somewhat excitable and anxious.

Danny's mother was concerned as she watched her neighbors across the street struggle with the unusual and distracted behaviors of their children, especially when it appeared that her son was following the same footsteps. She started to read everything she could get her hands on regarding autism and other developmental disorders. She reviewed current medical literature and programs used for dealing with autistic children. She began to implement some of the techniques that were currently boasting some success. Rapid changes, however, were not forthcoming. Her son could not speak, his comprehension of language was almost non-existent, and his behavior was bizarre. He required constant supervision and attention.

Danny's mother began investigating the avenue of heavy metal toxicities when she saw the sudden changes in the neighboring children's behavior and cognition. She also began to suspect that her child might have had excessive exposure to toxic metals as an infant.

Although the hair analysis result for her son did not appear to be terribly elevated in any particular metal (he did show low levels of lead, mercury, cadmium, arsenic, nickel, copper, and aluminum), provocative urine testing revealed more than five times the acceptable amount of lead was excreted from Danny's body. Keep in mind that this acceptable level is the same level used to evaluate toxicity in adults. Her child was only two years old and had a tiny body mass in comparison to an adult. Danny also excreted enormous quantities of copper; where an expected amount of copper excretion with provocation is somewhere between 2 and 36 μg/dl, her child had excreted 643 μg/dl. He also excreted seven times the acceptable level of nickel. Sudden, dramatic changes in Danny's agitated behavior and anxiety level occurred after excretion of these excessive toxic metals.

It's interesting to note that this little boy had his blood lead levels analyzed before commencing chelation. His blood lead was reported to be within the acceptable range. Unfortunately, the chronic exposure to lead and other metals was underestimated and underevaluated by the preliminary blood lead test. Bear in mind that the blood test revealed a moderately low amount of lead in the blood, which may well indicate an exposure that was present every day of this little boy's infancy. Danny's case demonstrates how lead can accumulate in the brain and nervous system, as well as other body tissues, while escaping detection. And other harmful metals, such as cadmium, aluminum, arsenic, mercury, and copper, are not even assessed by the blood testing procedure.

Danny's sister is also being tested for metal toxicity, though she is not showing overt symptoms, and Danny is making remarkable gains in growth and development.

Mrs. Simpson, a mother of two children diagnosed with autistic tendencies in Nova Scotia, heard about my children from her sister, a nurse, who had read an article I wrote for *Canadian Nurse* magazine describing my children's metal poisoning. Mrs. Simpson couldn't wait to talk with me. Not only did she have two children (boys aged four and six) who had been diagnosed with pervasive developmental disorder and autistic tendencies, but she remembered her family physician telling her something about "suspicious levels of lead" evident in her blood during a routine prenatal checkup before her second son was born. The importance of the blood lead evaluation hadn't registered at the time and her physician hadn't recommended any treatment or precautions. However, she was now consumed with worry. After reading current information pertaining to lead and other metal toxicities in children, she was certain that her children were victims of chronic metal accumulation.

Mrs. Simpson told me that what I had written about my own children described her children exactly. In fact, she said, it described almost one child in every block of her town in Nova Scotia, and many other children had more subtle problems that were suggestive of chronic metal burdens. She was frantic to have her own children tested. Within one week of our conversation, she had found a doctor who would use chelation to test her boys. Hair elemental analysis and provocative urine sampling results indicated excessive accumulation and excretion of heavy metals — lead, cadmium, arsenic, aluminum, copper. They also displayed a deficiency in lithium.

As chelation therapy relieved some of the accumulated body burden of toxic metals . . . you guessed it! The boys' behavior improved dramatically. Again, the improvements were witnessed by all working with the two children. And the doctor performing the testing and subsequent treatment was extremely surprised at the impressive results accompanying the detoxification of these children.

A friend of Mrs. Simpson had nine-year-old twin boys who were also diagnosed with autistic tendencies and pervasive developmental disorder. These twins began testing soon after Mrs. Simpson's children underwent treatment for excessive metal burden. They also demonstrated excessive metal burden and excretion patterns, and began to show improvements in their behavior and cognitive development almost immediately after the administration of chelation therapy and excretion of toxic metals. Both mothers are now passing this information on to other families of similarly disabled children.

Up to now I've been writing about young children, but I'd also like to tell you about some older children and teenagers affected by chronic metal toxicity, and then let Zigurts describe some adult patients he has dealt with in his practice.

During the course of our investigations, Zigurts and I began to suspect that if excessive metal exposure continued after infancy, a child would display gradually worsening symptoms, from more subtle signs like simple language delay and learning disabilities, to hyperactivity, attention deficit disorder, autism-like characteristics, and eventually profound mental retardation. We had been investigating younger children with autism-like characteristics when we suddenly recognized that there was an abundance of attention deficit disordered and learning disabled adolescents in our area. Because the research we had been reading stated in no uncertain terms that heavy metals can be responsible for these symptoms, we felt we had to investigate further.

Christopher Frost was a twelve-year-old child diagnosed at an early age with attention deficit disorder. He was prescribed Ritalin at age seven in an attempt to improve his concentration and attention. His behavior was bizarre. He was excessively hyperactive. He drove his parents nuts with his repetitive, useless, physical habits. He would ask the same questions over and over, or continue calling out your name after you had responded to him. He was a distraction in his class at school. Mrs. Frost had been called frequently by the school about things that Christopher had done wrong or not bothered to do at all, and now she was refusing to answer the school's calls. There was nothing satisfying about life with Christopher. It was damn difficult work trying to accommodate this child, and he had three siblings, all of them displaying similar types of disorders although none yet quite as drastic as his. Christopher's youngest brother had severe problems with language, cognitive development, and repetitive, compulsive behaviors. He had difficulty in socializing with his peers. The two middle children were not so difficult, but they also presented some minor attentional problems and lack of normal development.

The family's home was on a busy street in North Vancouver, one of the original streets in that area, built in the 1940s. It had undergone a lot of renovation as the children were growing up, but they had kept most of the original plumbing. Many of their neighbors were sick with chronic diseases of uncertain origin (lupus, cirrhosis of the liver, many cases of multiple sclerosis and chronic fatigue syndrome). All the evidence was beginning to add up. We had little doubt that some kind of environmental effect was disturbing normal bodily functions and causing chronic degenerative diseases.

All four Frost children were tested for heavy metal burden. All four displayed a combination of low to moderate levels of lead, cadmium, copper, aluminum, mercury, arsenic, and tin, but their *total* burden of metals far exceeded the acceptable guidelines, and the synergistic effects of some of the metal combinations would cause more cumulative, damaging effects. These children had almost no measurable manganese, an essential element that, in diminished concentrations, is known to cause disordered mental processes. Their lithium levels were also markedly depressed.

After these essential elements were replenished, chelation therapy was commenced. The amount of toxic metals these children excreted was phenomenal, and they have shown measurable improvements since. There is little doubt that metal poisoning was the underlying cause of their disorders. Even after treatment, however, Christopher has not been able to function successfully without his daily doses of Ritalin. Although some improvement has been observed in his behavior and cognitive functioning, we suspect that he has suffered permanent brain damage that, at this stage, may not be correctable.

The brain is a particularly remarkable body organ in its ability to compensate for injury, weakness, or disturbances. For example, after a serious injury to delicate brain tissues, other areas of the brain can be retrained to compensate or provide some of the functions that the damaged portion was previously responsible for. There have been many cases of incredible rehabilitation of brain function in adults with brain damage. As young children are continuing to grow and expand their own resources and experiences, it is likely that there is more chance of brain retraining in a child.

Even with the brain's adaptability, many researchers report findings of permanent brain damage in chronically toxic children. The Ruff/Bijur study mentioned in Chapter 4 suggested that structural and functional changes occur in brain tissue from lead deposition. This makes me think that some of the successful changes we are witnessing after chelation treatment could be a result of functional improvement, perhaps an improvement in neurotransmitter functions. At the same time, when we see less change it could indicate permanent structural damage of important cell components. This distinction between structural and functional damage would also account for the dramatic improvements, but no complete recoveries in any of these children, including my own.

Another victim of attention deficit disorder and severe learning disabilities, Michael Wilson was an eleven-year-old child who had used Ritalin since age seven to help improve his concentration and attention span. Michael had been impulsive and a big distraction ever since he was a young child, and his parents were devastated that his functioning continued to lag behind that of his peers. It appeared that Michael had reached his saturation point, that he was unable to comprehend school work at the Grade 5 level. It wasn't that he didn't try, he just couldn't do the work even though he seemed to be a bright child. Consequently, he was frustrated and his self-esteem was deflating. He was sent to special classes for the learning disabled. He had no real friends. He was not invited over to play with other children after school because of his over-zealous activity, disturbing impulsiveness, and general immaturity.

When they learned about the effects of metal toxicity, his family was eager to begin testing for heavy metal burden. Sure enough, Michael turned out to be yet another child suffering from the toxic effects of heavy metals. His results indicated an enormous amount of cadmium, lead, arsenic, tin, and aluminum. Elemental deficiencies were also noted, and supplemented before chelation therapy began. He continued to expel huge quantities of toxic metals through several courses of chelation therapy. His attention span improved slightly during this time. He, himself, felt that he could concentrate better. Although he continues to depend on the Ritalin therapy, he is making significant gains. And although time will tell more of a story for this young boy, this does lead us to believe that early detection and removal of excessive metal burden are critical for the best results.

Phil Johal, a thirteen-year-old boy, was excitable, terribly impulsive, a distraction in class and at home, and was doing poorly in school. It was not that he was incapable of doing the work; he could not stay on task in order to complete any project. He could not sit still. His mind was going a hundred miles an hour. He couldn't control himself. Phil was always in trouble.

He presented some other unusual problems. He was photophobic and could not stay in a well-lit room for any length of time. At home he preferred to be in darkness — his blinds were always pulled. The light hurt his eyes and made him feel unwell. His clothes bothered him. Anything tight drove him to distraction. He had to wear loose-fitting clothing because fabric irritated his skin.

When the possibility that Phil was metal toxic was suggested, his mother remembered that, as a youngster, Phil had all of the gastric symptoms of metal toxicity. She also said that she had always tasted a metallic flavor in her mouth during Phil's early infancy.

Phil's first treatment of oral chelation didn't reveal excessive metal excretion. However, his hair elemental analysis indicated extreme metal burden. Another oral chelating agent was prescribed and, lo and behold, huge quantities of toxic metals began to spill. This suggests another important factor. Some people seem to have toxic metals bound in a pattern that's much more difficult to disrupt. The original oral chelator that was prescribed, Cuprimine, worked extremely well for the majority of younger children that we had been observing. But it didn't work in Phil's case. Instead, DMSA proved to be more efficient. Body burden testing of Phil revealed tremendous amounts of cadmium. He also displayed a large concentration of lead and aluminum. His lithium levels appeared to be extremely depressed.

Phil is now performing well at school; his teachers have noticed an improvement and Phil himself feels that he is far more capable of concentrating. He no longer needs to be immersed in darkness and his clothes do not bother him as before. His complexion, previously pasty and pale, has dramatically improved — perhaps he was another victim of toxic metal anemia. Phil is far less agitated, excitable, and impulsive than before. His actions are spent generally on functional body movement rather than repetitive, useless motion. His ability to stay on task has improved. He is now able to complete more of his school work on time.

Sean Gerard, diagnosed with extreme attention deficit disorder and hyperactivity, was also the victim of a severe hearing impairment. For no explainable reason he had lost most of his hearing in one ear. He was using a hearing aid at age nine. He was a chronic disrupter in class, was terribly impulsive, and drove his family crazy. The Gerards couldn't understand his bizarre, uncontrollable behavior. It was upsetting and embarrassing, and Sean was losing his ability to function in a classroom setting.

Sean was almost always agitated and anxious. He had periods of great emotional upset and turmoil. It broke his mother's heart to see what was happening to her son. It made her feel even more uneasy after recognizing that Sean might be suffering from the effects of chronic metal toxicity, especially when she remembered that, during Sean's infancy, they had done a complete renovation of their old home — while they were living in it. They had consumed water right from the tap first thing in the morning and used it for preparing infant formula. As an infant, Sean had displayed all of the gastric symptoms of toxic metal exposure. Mrs. Gerard had often taken him to the doctor's office to try to get to the bottom of his constant crying episodes, agitation, colic, and anxiety. Never had anyone suggested checking for heavy metal ingestion. His mother now clearly recognized that, as a baby, Sean had been exposed to the majority of sources known to cause metal toxicity.

Sean has just recently been tested for body burden of toxic metals. Preliminary results indicate a huge concentration of cadmium in his body tissues.

These are only a few of the children we have been observing over the last eighteen months. Their stories are all surprisingly similar — as are the majority of improvements noted to date. Therefore, for fear of boring readers, we have not dwelled on each piece of clinical success and we will now move on. Since we began these investigations, many more parents have contacted us — the case studies alone could fill a book. We have also observed a few children with excessive metal burden who have not responded as dramatically as the children we have described. Some have not appeared to improve at all. And some children with similar diagnoses have not tested positive for excessive metal burden. Toxicity is not always the answer. There are other factors which can also cause these disorders. Genetic causes, chemical imbalances, non-metal environmental toxins, viruses, auto-immune responses, and physical injuries can also damage delicate areas of brain tissue. Similar symptoms indicate only that the same portion of the brain has been damaged. (For more information about autism and attention deficit disorder, their characteristics, causes, and diagnosing, please see the Appendix.)

Now let's consider the big children — adults! Adults can also be exposed to excessive heavy metals and, when suffering the effects of chronic toxicity, they also commonly escape medical detection. During the last decade, Zigurts has gained a huge appreciation for the insidious, severe, and extremely debilitating damage that these metals inflict upon us. On the next few pages he relates some of his personal case studies, and in the next chapter he tells his own family's story.

In my medical practice, I have had many experiences with adults affected by chronic metal toxicity. One of my patients, a 36-year-old businessman with a history of gout and hypertension, came to see me several years ago complaining of acute gouty arthritis of the big toe. I treated him in the conventional manner with diet modification, weight loss, and medication. Despite these efforts, his uric acid levels remained at the high range of normal and tended to slip into the toxic or symptomatic range periodically. His blood pressure remained unstable. I assumed he was under a great deal of stress because of his business and therefore advised him to undertake an exercise program to help work off some of his anxiety and to improve his cardiovascular status. He managed to lose considerable weight and his blood pressure did come down somewhat but still remained too high. One day he asked me about chelation therapy and we discussed what benefit there might be in screening him for heavy metal toxicity. Significant in his history was that he owned a delivery service and spent a lot of time in traffic where lead exposure was relatively high.

Preliminary hair elemental analysis showed lead levels of 26.1 parts per million where 5 or 6 parts per million are suggestive of lead toxicity. Urine testing further supported this finding. The patient was chelated with a course of intravenous EDTA. After about ten treatments, his wife reported that he seemed much less anxious and irritable, he was able to sleep better, and had considerably more energy — work did not take all that he had. In addition, his uric acid levels dropped into the normal range; his kidney function had obviously improved.

A second case involved a 55-year-old gas station owner-operator, who had been in the business for approximately 40 years. In 1985 he developed colicky abdominal pains for which he was thoroughly investigated but no diagnosis was ever made. Five years later he developed symptoms of angina. He was admitted to a coronary care unit for monitoring after a couple of acute episodes of chest pain. Tests did not reveal any cardiac damage and his coronary vessels were not appreciably blocked.

About a year later, following a root canal and extraction procedure, this man developed facial pains and swelling, and occasionally felt a discharge of purulent material into the back of his throat. He subsequently was operated on for a mastoiditis or infection of the mastoid bone behind his ear. Despite extensive investigations and procedures, the foul-tasting sensation of discharge in the back of his throat persisted.

A year after the dental work, this man began to have seizures. It was thought that the sensation of drainage in the back of his throat was actually a pre-seizure "aura." He was placed on anti-seizure medications, but despite this he developed a seizure disorder which meant he had generalized seizures once and sometimes twice a week.

This fellow was a friend of my father's and had repaired

all of our family vehicles at one time or another. On hearing about this history, I suggested that perhaps he should consider being tested for heavy metal toxicity. His family physician apparently did do a blood test, and the lead level was found to be within the high normal range. In addition, this man had three additional molars removed. There was temporary relief, but then the sensation of discharge in the back of his throat returned.

A few months later I received an emergency call to this man's garage — he was having some kind of attack and refused to be taken to hospital. I found the man sitting hunched over in a vehicle, slurring his speech, complaining of chest pain, and looking as if he might lose consciousness at any moment. I quickly summoned an ambulance and stretched him out on the ground, testing his pulse and blood pressure which were both normal.

After the emergency response team arrived, stabilized him, and transported him to hospital, I told the family that I suspected a heart attack but was not entirely sure. Apparently he had had similar episodes previously and no sign of any cardiac involvement was found. In this instance, the hospital again found no cardiac abnormalities and released the man the next day. I advised him to come and see me about lead toxicity.

His hair lead levels were 436 parts per million, and provocative urine testing with EDTA revealed elevated arsenic and lead levels to confirm the diagnosis.

After five or six treatments, the patient did not feel the symptoms of grogginess that preceded seizures, nor did he have any more seizures. About two weeks after his first treatment he discontinued his seizure medications and has not looked back. He also has not had any problems with chest discomfort or the abdominal colicky pains which occurred frequently.

For a minute, think back to the first child we spoke of — Bobby Smith. Bobby had abdominal pain and seizures. As previously mentioned, when excessive lead is ingested it can cause gut symptoms. When excessive lead is deposited in brain tissues, it can cause seizures. Lead can also cause changes in cardiac status, even cardiac irregularities.

Because of my suspicion of immune system deficiency due to chronic toxicity, and what appeared to be the development of draining cavitations in his jaws, I sent him to a dentist. Dental surgery revealed incompletely healed cavities in the jaw bones where the extracted teeth had been located. Residual tissue was cleaned out and the patient has not suffered from any more swelling and sensations of discharge into his throat.

My last case involves a 60-year-old man who ran a cleaning business and had become disabled because of unstable angina due to coronary and aortic valve disease. In 1987 he had surgery for an aortic aneurysm which was accidentally sutured to his chest wall. As his coronary and aortic valve disease progressively worsened, he developed atherosclerotic blockages and became a high risk patient for open heart surgery. He was therefore treated with two angioplasties, the second of which was unsuccessful. He subsequently deteriorated and there was nothing that could be done for him. The patient complained of symptoms of decreased exercise tolerance, severe fatigue, angina at rest, a dizzy, foggy feeling, and hazy vision that appeared to be deteriorating. He also had hypertension.

Provocative urine testing showed increased levels of aluminum, arsenic, and lead. By the time he finished 30 treatments, he was able to return to work. He no longer had any chest pains and his vision had cleared up. Where his blood pressure was as high as 190/95, it stabilized around 150/80. He also commented, in front of his blushing wife, that his sexual functioning had returned.

Consider again the signs and symptoms of acute and chronic lead poisoning. In both the child and the adult, colicky abdominal pain can be an initial symptom. Both children and adults may show pallor caused by anemia, and may experience fatigue, listlessness or irritability, muscle and joint aches and pains, wrist drop or foot drop, tremulousness, headaches, and slurring of speech. When symptoms are severe, acute kidney failure, convulsions, coma, and death may occur.

Chronically exposed patients may develop some of the above signs very gradually as body burden of lead accumulates. They may have normal blood lead levels and perhaps normal hair lead levels if exposure and accumulation have been gradual enough. In extreme circumstances, where exposure has been extremely gradual or where the last exposure occurred six months to a year earlier, the only hope for detecting high levels of lead would be with a provocative urine test.

There may be considerable overlap between acute and chronic signs of lead poisoning. There may be underlying chronic signs because of an accumulation in body burden of lead with superimposed signs of acute toxicity due to episodes of more rapid accumulation or increased sensitivity due to decreased tolerance for further accumulations of heavy metal.

Note that subtle signs of abdominal colic, fatigue, or attention and memory deficits may be the only clues. These symptoms can occur with numerous other illnesses. It is therefore not uncommon for patients to undergo extensive investigations without obtaining a definitive diagnosis because lead poisoning is not considered or, when it is, the appropriate tests are not done.

Note that in our patient with a ten-year history of abdominal colicky pain, a five-year history of cardiovascular symptoms, and a more recent history of immune compromise and a seizure disorder, it took ten years to consider lead poisoning as a potential cause. Blood lead level was within normal range but hair lead levels were 100 times above normal and provocative urine testing showed excess elimination of lead.

Our younger patient with symptoms of irritability, fatigue, changes in concentration, hypertension and gout also turned up high levels of lead.

The important part of these individuals' presentation was their history. Both had been exposed to high levels of lead due to their work in the automotive industry and due to spending a lot of time in urban traffic. The last patient had a history of exposure to cleaning agents, many of which contain toxic metals.

Biologically and physiologically the only difference between adults and children is that children have a higher metabolic rate and tend to be more sensitive to lead toxicity. The cases presented show that history can be important, but in the absence of a clear incident of exposure to metals, one should still consider heavy metal poisoning based on the clinical presentation.

When addressing our personal observations of children and adults suffering the effects of chronic metal toxicity, many physicians will argue that we have provided only anecdotal evidence — not controlled, double-blind studies. And they are right. However, until a qualified medical body has the resources, finances, energy, and interest to complete the necessary controlled studies which must be done and which would take, incidentally, eight to ten years to complete, this book is likely the best that medicine has got right now. And, when I reflect on the damage to the young children in our case studies, I know that carefully researched and documented information already compiled by reputable medical bodies informs us this is precisely what we could have expected to happen to young developing children. The research has already been done. Let's use it.

8

Serendipity —
A Mother of Invention

Have you ever noticed that when you are desperate, when
you want something badly and you are trying as hard as you
can, nothing happens? And then, just as you are ready to
give up — you have capitulated, perhaps you still have the
occasional dream of hope but you are half-way to quitting
— just then things spontaneously fall into place. Some
would argue that necessity is the mother of invention but in
a case like this I think serendipity is.

As a new physician I didn't worry much about serendipity
ten years ago as I raced around the city in the middle of the
night in my red GTS with five-speed transmission and extra
wide tires, doing house calls to augment my income while
I was raising my young family and building my new medical
practice. I had to have a good car radio so I could listen to
Pat Burns, the local talk-show host who came on the air
when normal people went to sleep and there were only the
insomniacs, the taxi drivers, and me listening. Several times
I heard patients call in to discuss chelation therapy as a
means of treating cardiovascular disease. Little did I know
that this was an introduction to a treatment which would
eventually change the lives of Brett and Cameron Hallaway,
and the lives of many others, including my own son.

At the time I had just moved with my wife, our infant son,
and our dog into a new home in a wooded area. It was in a
valley with one main highway a few blocks away and an-

other main highway about a mile away on the other side of our property. Our house was built on the oldest foundation in the area with some additions added within the previous ten years that made it look rather modern. Within a short time of moving in, we did what every young family in an older house does, we started remodelling. This involved scraping, heating, and peeling paint, knocking down walls, stripping down old plaster to replace it with modern gypboard. There was dust everywhere, lead dust. But we didn't know. Our little boy was just pushing those toys around through the house, crawling on his hands and knees, doing all the things that kids normally do when they're two years old. Other than tell him to stay away from the dust, we didn't think there was too much to be concerned with.

Over the next few years I had forgotten about chelation therapy until one of my back-pain patients came to my office, pale as a ghost, huffing and puffing. I knew something was seriously wrong as he looked very frightened. He was 40 years of age and had just had a massive heart attack. He couldn't walk 25 feet without stopping for breath. He was diagnosed with severe blockages of four coronary arteries and had been told that he was not a candidate for surgery because of the severity of his disease. He was told to get his affairs in order.

After reviewing his medications and looking at his management, I could add nothing to what was being done. He was getting the best treatment available but was still facing the prospect of death. Then I remembered Pat Burns on his radio show speaking about chelation therapy. I suggested to the patient that he investigate this avenue as there was nothing else available to him. He ended up going to Bellingham, Washington, for treatment, and by the time he had completed twenty treatments he was walking three miles! After further treatments he was able to return to work. This was six years ago. He is still alive and has no symptoms of angina.

A fellow physician who was also my patient came to the

same crossroads in 1990. He had to go on medical disability because of coronary artery disease and angina with minimal exertion. He was not going to have surgery under any circumstances, so I told him the story of my other patient who had done so well. Although he sounded skeptical at first, eventually he attended a public meeting and did some research. He started chelation therapy and was soon well enough to return to working full days, sometimes six days per week. Eventually we both attended a training course put on by the American College for Advancement in Medicine and started using chelation therapy for our patients. We soon found that patients experienced relief of many symptoms including fatigue, arthritic pains, visual disturbances due to cataract opacities, insomnia, cool extremities, etc.

Despite acquiring this new interest, I continued on with my family practice, much of which had to do with the treatment of musculoskeletal injuries. That is how I met Nancy Hallaway. During our first appointment I observed an anxious mother with her life complicated by back pain. I could see that her thoughts were elsewhere. The sooner we could be finished, the sooner she could leave. Because of this impatience, I became curious. At that point I found out that she had two boys who were mentally handicapped and had been diagnosed as autistic.

My understanding of autism was that it was a permanent disability with severe neurological dysfunction. I felt sorry for the woman when she tried to describe how unmanageable these children were and how difficult it was to leave them with a babysitter. I naively invited her to bring them with her next time and she again tried to emphasize the reality and consequences of bringing her children with her. She said to me, "They'd be bouncing off your walls . . . they'd eat your walls. I'm serious."

I thought, "Aha! Pica." Pica is a disorder that is prevalent among children with heavy metal toxicity, or suffering from trace mineral deficiencies.

I became more curious. On further questioning I found that the family had lived in an old house which they had remodelled while the twins were infants. I also found out that they had appeared normal at birth and showed normal sucking behavior, normal eye contact, and interaction with parents for approximately the first year. The remodelling seemed to coincide with the time that these children began to show signs of deterioration.

I had recently attended a meeting of the American College for Advancement in Medicine and listened to a couple of lectures that dealt with environmental toxicity, including heavy metal toxicity, and the risks for children. It all seemed to fall into place and I told my patient what my thoughts were — with some reservation, as I had not treated children for heavy metal toxicity before this encounter.

Upon my insistence and perhaps to show me how ridiculous I was, Nancy decided to bring one of her children to my office so I could appreciate why it was not such a good idea.

I was not able to examine this child when they did come in. I don't think he sat still for more than 30 seconds. He was totally distracted and did not even notice my presence. We could not give him any commands. It was all I could do to speak to Nancy as we both chased after the boy in the closed room as he randomly selected various instruments and containers to drop, to chew, or to do whatever with or on. I quickly gained an appreciation for her plight and acknowledged that she was entirely right in finding someone else to look after her kids so that she could come back in and we could talk. We went on to test these children and treat them, and the rest is history.

Shortly after the Hallaway boys were treated, I realized that there was a possibility that my oldest son, who was having severe difficulty learning, could also be suffering from metal poisoning. I suddenly began to remember all of the dust that was around when we remodelled our house, all of the soldered copper plumbing, and all of the pollution that was in our yard and in our house from the two bordering highways.

At this point we had moved again, primarily to get away from the pollution associated with urban metropolitan life. We had escaped to the burbs. What a place — creek in the back yard, trees, long winding driveway, a big tree with a rope to swing across the creek, and a park with tennis courts on the other side of the creek. But all was not so well. Many evenings my wife and I would try to help my son with his reading and with his preschool and schoolwork. I recalled how frustrated we were when we taught him the first word of a sentence and by the time he had learned the second word, he had forgotten the first one. We struggled for hours reading one paragraph. I was worried. I could see that his academic capacity was such that he would be lucky to graduate from high school. We would push and try so hard that my son would break down into tears and, inside, so would I.

My parents thought that it was poor parenting, that we were not spending enough time teaching the children how to read. They did not seem to understand when I told them we were spending plenty of time teaching them and there might be something more seriously wrong. I recall one occasion when, in an attempt to stop the criticism, I retorted that it was probably a genetic deficiency that had been inherited from our side of the family. There was a moment of shock, and an uncomfortable silence as my father realized that, however remote the possibility, it might be true. I can't recall him saying anything except a subdued goodbye as he walked out of the house.

This kind of thing affects the entire family. We spent so much time with this child that we felt guilty that we were depriving the other children of contact that they needed. We eventually took him to a private learning centre for an evaluation and found out that, although he was in Grade 4, his reading skills were at the Grade 2 level.

It was not until we took him for testing at the private center that his public school teacher took notice and ordered tests to be run through the school board, evaluating his learning skills. We would have to wait a year before they would be able to book him in for tests, so we decided to send him to the private learning center in addition to attending school. He went for one hour, three times a week.

It was costing us a bundle of money, but he was moving forward, however slowly, and he was not having to suffer the tears and sorrow trying to live up to the expectations that he knew we had of him regardless of how hard we tried to hide them. Sometimes our frustrations would just come through. At times we thought he was lazy, that he wasn't listening, that he didn't want to learn.

On one occasion I noticed that he had a lateral squint — one of his eyes deviated outward. I almost cheered with relief because I assumed that his gaze problem was responsible for his learning difficulties. We sent him to an ophthalmologist who prescribed eye exercises. We had him perform these religiously and the strabismus disappeared unless he got tired in the evenings watching television or trying to read.

It was after I had tested and treated the Hallaway twins, and after we had obtained such tremendous results, that the idea struck me that perhaps my own child was metal poisoned; after all, gaze defects of the eyes could be attributable to heavy metals, in particular aluminum. So I tested my son and found that he had an excess of copper, an excess of lead, and had very high levels, toxic levels of aluminum. In his urine he even dumped arsenic and cadmium. Where on earth did he pick all that crap up? Was it coming from the pop cans, from the plumbing where we had lived? Regardless, he needed treatment.

A short time after commencing treatment, I saw that he was clearing up. Before we finished the provocative testing I noticed a change in his reading ability. He seemed much more focused. He no longer complained of fatigue of his eyes. I gave him two more bouts of treatment and found that he continued to improve with each successive course of therapy. His marks in school gradually started to come up and he is now at the Grade 6 level with As and Bs in math and science and C+s in his English. He is a changed young man who has no difficulty with recall and/or concentration. The insecurities, the uncertainties, and the tears are no longer present.

9

Where Is the Stuff Coming From?

Lead does not fulfill any necessary function in the human body. It was never intended to be in the human body and shouldn't be in it . . . period.

In its natural state, lead, a heavy metal of bluish color that is pliable, inelastic, and easily fusible, poses no problems to living organisms as it lies in the earth's crust. Lead generally occurs in ores combined with silver, zinc, copper, arsenic, antimony, or bismuth. Lead forms many salts (compounds produced by the combination of a base with an acid), oxides (the combination of an element with oxygen), and organometallic compounds (mixtures of metal and carbon compounds). Lead's affinity for other metals makes it useful to industry. And it was a particularly exciting metal for alchemists who believed lead could be transformed into gold. We believe we've finally found the only way to transform lead into gold.

Lead is possibly the oldest metal known to man — the earliest archaeological evidence of its use dates back to 3000 BC. The ancient Greeks were probably the first to expose lead to the earth's surface in their search for silver deposits. Lead eventually became an important commodity in its own right, but once lead deposits began to be mined, the toxic effects of lead began to surface. For example, the metal was used in wine-making. As long-term storage often resulted in a putrid-tasting product, Greek vintners boiled wine in large vats made of pure lead to better preserve it. The lead leached out into the finished product. These wine-making practices may have killed putrefying bacteria but they greatly increased human exposure to lead, particularly in cultures along the shores of the Mediterranean.

Later the Romans adopted some of the Greek wine-making practices, and also developed a sweetened grape concentrate that was stored in lead decanters. An ounce or two of this concentrate was added to a goblet of wine to sweeten the flavor. Just one thimble of sweetener had enough lead in it to render one of us lead toxic were we to imbibe, and the average aristocrat consumed perhaps a litre or two of wine daily. Lead was also used to line Roman aqueducts, the marvelous water networks that brought water into their cities and distributed it to their homes. They also coated copper tableware with lead to avoid the metallic taste of copper. Using lead to transport and store water, process wine, and serve food, caused chronic, widespread lead toxicity. It has been suggested by historians that copper/lead poisoning may have been a major factor in the fall of the Roman Empire.

Lead was one of the first metals to be mined in North America. It was used primarily by the early European settlers for making shot. Of course, mining lead ore in North America eventually resulted in increasing levels of environmental contamination and human exposure. As industrialization of our earth has expanded, it is no wonder that we face a huge environmental health crisis. And I am focusing only on lead.

The Soviet Union was the world's largest producer of lead until it broke up. Now Australia ranks as the top producer with the United States second. Canada is another major source of lead and lead ore is also mined extensively in Mexico, Peru, Yugoslavia, Germany, Morocco, Southwest Africa, and Spain. However, no country is exempt from the use of lead products or from the potential health hazards of excessive lead exposure.

It has been estimated that the world continues to mine about 6 million tons of lead every year. Lead production in the United States has more than doubled since the 1960s; more than 400,000 tons are mined annually, and the country consumes approximately 50 percent of the world's production of lead. The New York-based Lead Industries Association estimates that approximately 90 percent of American products containing lead are recycled. The association reported that 800,000 tons of lead were reclaimed by secondary smelters in 1988. The large majority of this lead came from recycling automobile batteries. Smelters which process lead ore, and the secondary smelters which recover the metal from recycled batteries and other products, emit high concentrations of airborne lead particles. These facts and figures help substantiate the claim that there has been an increase of lead in the atmosphere. And quite simply, lead does not belong above the earth's crust.

Today, lead is used mostly in the production of large storage batteries. It is estimated that about 80 percent of all lead consumed in the United States goes into storage batteries designed for automobiles, trucks, and boats. It is also used in lead-acid batteries which power electric vehicles (*i.e.*, forklifts, wheelchairs, golf carts, and the newer electric cars built to replace gasoline-powered cars). Other industrial uses of lead include soldering materials for electronic circuitboards, cable coverings, construction materials, pigments (in paints, plastics, etc.), solder, ammunition, primer coatings for automobiles, ceramics, weights, paints for bridges, roadmarkings, and industrial equipment. Lead arsenates have been popular in past years and have been used in vast quantities as insecticides for crop protection.

How does this relate to children? Children are exposed to lead in various ways. Particles of lead can be inhaled or swallowed. They can be found in air that may look clean. They can be found in food and water. They can be found in our homes and in our yards.

Lead is commonly found in house dust. Lead paint dust can rub or chip off walls, windows, doors, etc. Although lead was banned from interior paints in 1978, it's still allowed in exterior paints. Approximately 75 percent of homes built before 1980 are covered with lead paint. There are over 50 million homes in the United States that have lead-based paint on exterior and interior walls. This paint may be covered with one or two layers of newer paint and possibly wallpaper. Nonetheless, it's there and when it's disturbed during remodelling or sanding, the dust produced becomes a hazard. Renovations of houses with older paint or other lead products can stir up a whole heap of trouble for young children. Children inhale and ingest lead dust. As toddlers spend so much of their early lives playing and crawling around on the ground and putting their hands into their mouths, they pick it up from many different sources: their fingers, their toys, their clothes, to name a few.

The U.S. Environmental Protection Agency (EPA) estimates that drinking water is the source of 10 to 20 percent of lead exposure for children. They estimate that approximately 20 percent of the population is exposed to levels of lead in their water which produce a drastic increase of lead levels in a child's blood. Water supplies can be contaminated from atmospheric and ground sources, and lead can also leach out of water mains and household plumbing. In North America, many pipes and water ducts from the turn of the century were solid lead. More recently, pipes were made of copper soldered with lead-based solders. With the acidification of our atmospheric moisture and rain, water in reservoirs has become acidified and as it travels through these old pipes and water ducts it absorbs whatever metals it comes in contact with. Lead is found in most water supplies in varying amounts. After travelling through our water mains and household plumbing it is often found in exceedingly high concentrations, particularly in the first morning draw of tap water (or any draw of tap water which has been sitting in the pipes for any significant length of time). Never, ever use this first draw of water, especially in mixing baby formula or other fluids to feed to your kids. Infants who drink formula mixed with tap water that is contaminated with lead are extremely susceptible and vulnerable to accidental lead poisoning.

It has only been in recent years that lead solder was banned from the plumbing industry — because they found out that it was potentially harmful to our health. But the lead used to solder the water mains that were put in decades ago is still there. When water is highly acidic — and water polluted by "acid rain" does become acidic — it causes more lead, copper, and other metals to be ionized out or brought into solution. The majority of homes still have copper water pipes with lead solder. Think about it. What do you see deposited around the drain under a leaky faucet? That green stain is copper that has leached into your drinking water.

Banning lead from water pipes has changed but not ended the problem. With the decreased use of lead solder and pipes, and the reliance on polyvinyl chloride (PVC) materials, we have introduced a new contaminant, cadmium, which is used as a stabilizer for PVC resins. (Lead is also used in some PVC resins as a stabilizer.) There is less metal available to the water running through these pipes compared to the older pipes. With the increased use of PVC piping the amount of lead in drinking water may have decreased but the amount of lead in the atmosphere has continued to increase.

Our children are exposed to lead in the air. During the leaded gasoline era, the amount of lead emitted into the atmosphere as a result of combustion of fossil fuels was in excess of 100,000 tons. Research indicates that 40 to 50 percent of lead that we breathe is ultimately absorbed by our bodies.

Car emissions which previously saturated our city air from many decades of leaded gasoline use have caused incredible pollution and contamination. Airborne lead particles are extremely small, less than 1 micron (one one-thousandth of a millimetre) in diameter, and do not readily fall out of the sky. Thus, these lead particles remain in the air for months, even years.

It has been suggested that in cities with excessive traffic volume, 90 percent of airborne lead from the 1970s to 1980s came from car exhaust. The type of lead additive used in gasoline was tetraethyl lead, a supertoxic form of lead. Although tetraethyl lead is mostly discharged from tailpipes as less toxic lead compounds, a significant amount remains in the form of tetraethyl lead. It's no wonder that lead additives are being banned from gasoline. Governments from many countries now verify that, since the discontinuation of lead additives in gasoline, city children's blood levels have shown a significant drop from the years in which leaded gasoline was so popular. Leaded gasoline is next to impossible to find in Canada. On the other hand, developing countries have not established the stringent controls that are being established in North America, and you can still buy leaded gasoline in many places around the world including the United States (though it's less available than it was five years ago) and Mexico.

Car lead emissions cause air pollution but they also contaminate the soil and water near major roadways. The soil of high-volume traffic areas has been contaminated by many decades of emissions. In the United States, many studies have revealed that some of these well-travelled roadways are bordered by contaminated soil up to a mile from the road. These areas, which often exceed the federal lead-pollution guidelines and standards for hazardous waste sites, may include playgrounds, sidewalks, your back yard, or your children's sandbox.

Coal burning produces a significant amount of atmospheric lead, and incineration of municipal garbage, highly acclaimed as an answer to overflowing landfills as it reduces the visible evidence of excessive waste, is a new source of airborne lead. In 1992 an estimated 50,000 tons of lead were discarded. A large proportion of this is subjected to high-temperature burning which can vaporize lead and spread it throughout the environment. Lead is also melted down and frequently there is no control of the vapors that are emitted as lead reaches its melting point.

Once lead is in the atmosphere or in the soil it does not just go away and disappear. All of these lead emissions remain in the dirt and dust until they are removed. And who's removing them? No one! Unfortunately, the cost of removing lead is enormous. Removal has been and probably always will be the focus of an on-going, heated debate among health officials, lead producers, car manufacturers, government officials and, increasingly, an informed public — you and me.

Lead can be found in the food we eat that has unknowingly been grown in contaminated soil or irrigated by contaminated water. Plants incorporate lead just as humans do by absorbing contaminated water and soil. Fish and shellfish are high on the list of potentially contaminated food as they ingest waterborne lead. Until the late 1970s, lead was commonly used as the soldering material for canned foods. Yes, even for infant formula! This was previously a common source of lead exposure for children as the lead would leach into the formula from the can. Lead and other heavy metal leaching can still be a problem in cans which contain acidic fluids. For example, have you ever looked at the chemical reaction that takes place on the metal inside a can of tomato juice? Despite the lead soldering ban in America, some countries still refuse to outlaw its use in canning, so lead can be found in some cans of imported foods. You can identify these cans by the outraised line along the seam.

Recently we heard of a case where a child being poisoned by water that was boiled in a kettle that had been imported from the Middle East. This kettle's joints were soldered with lead solder.

Other sources of lead that are less likely to affect children but could poison adults are industrial uses. The automotive industry is still a source of considerable contamination as lead is used in some fuels and lubricants, and to solder leaks and joints in radiators.

Anyone involved in demolition or in the scrap metal business is at significant risk. As bridges, other steel structures, homes, and buildings are demolished, lead content is mobilized. Sandblasting to remove old paint is a major source of contamination. Individuals doing this type of work should be well protected, and some attempt should be made to keep the resulting dust from being carried far afield from the worksite.

One of the worst areas of industrial activity is in the lead storage battery manufacture and recycling industry. Lead is found in the acidified solution of these batteries and how these battery acids are disposed of is anyone's guess. Frequently they are just dumped onto the ground or into a sewer drain. The lead then enters our water systems and affects well water, or enters streams and rivers to contaminate the food chain.

Linoleum and putty contain significant amounts of lead. There are still paint pigments and anti-foulants that contain lead. Some lead is used as sheathing for wire cables. Both manufacturers and users of these cables are at risk of contamination.

Jewelers working with lead are at risk, as are potters. Glazes in pottery and dishes often contain lead. One should always buy pottery that is labelled "lead-free."

There's considerable risk of lead exposure for shooters at target ranges. Recently we saw a young child with lead poisoning whose mother and father were both avid target shooters. The child had picked up lead from their hands, clothing, and their discharged ammunition casings.

Other heavy metals

Obviously, lead is not the only heavy metal that can account for neurological compromise and other negative health effects. It has been the glamour metal of the last few decades, receiving much publicity from the media and much attention from scientists. Its effects are the most well researched and documented of the heavy metal group of elements. Other metals haven't been that well scrutinized yet.

You will have noticed throughout this book that heavy metals (a group of elements identified by their peculiar luster, fusibility, malleability, and ability to conduct heat and electricity) have been referred to as being extremely toxic. During particular stages of human development these metals will cause dysfunction and may cause irreversible damage, especially when they affect the immature brain and nervous system. The United States Council of Environmental Quality as far back as 1976 deemed fourteen metals to be extremely hazardous to human life and the environment. These metals are arsenic, barium, beryllium, cadmium, chromium, copper, lead, manganese, mercury, nickel, selenium, silver, vanadium, and zinc. The EPA noted the five most dangerous air pollutants to be, in order of importance, cadmium, lead, nickel, beryllium, and antimony. Long-term exposure to any of these metals will produce irreparable damage to body cells, tissues, and organs.

The effects of toxic metals are similar in that they all will cause neurological damage, tissue damage, and kidney and liver problems if not removed. They can all accumulate in toxic amounts in a child's body due to the rapid rate of metabolism of the developing child. These metals alone or in combination with other heavy metals can be responsible for gross neurological problems in children. When it comes to heavy metal and mineral imbalances, lead, mercury, arsenic, cadmium, and aluminum have been clearly identified as causing intellectual impairment. Manganese, copper, and tin have also been implicated.

An important consideration is the combination of lead and other toxins. There is increasing evidence suggesting that specific combinations of metals have synergistic effects that are responsible for compounding the more severe problems in children. This means that a combination of two or more metals can be many times more toxic than the expected sum of toxicity of the metals.

To further complicate matters, the presence of heavy metals in body tissues can cause dysfunctional cellular enzyme activity and nutritional absorption problems which lead to nutritional deficiencies and the depletion of essential elements. A child's body becomes transformed from a healthy living entity into a toxic chemical cesspool. No wonder these young children, when left undiagnosed, misdiagnosed, and untreated, are experiencing such an incredible degree of neurological dysfunction and cerebral irritation.

The further you look into heavy metals and their toxic effects on young children, the more you begin to realize that virtually all metals can be neurotoxic. Although some are deemed to be essential elements and are required in certain quantities for proper bodily functioning, even these can be toxic if present in excess quantities. The non-essential metals have no known purpose or function in human tissues. They should not be in there at all. Each metal ion in this category will cause damage to the body cell that it is sequestered in. These are substances that we are not naturally born with in our bodies (unless of course these toxins have passed through the placenta from our mothers) but research indicates that many of these non-essential elements are commonly found in our bodies today. There are even acceptable levels of these toxins that are presumed to be relatively safe but these levels were only established because the existing technology was unable to measure any smaller amounts. As technology improved, the safe body burden of metals has been set lower. Research is showing that many of these new low limits are not as harmless as was once thought. Science is demonstrating that damage occurs to body tissues at levels lower than those claimed to be safe.

The following section lists the most toxic non-essential and essential elements with a brief description of their effects and their sources.

NON-ESSENTIAL TRACE ELEMENTS

Cadmium

Cadmium is one "bad-ass," supertoxic heavy metal. It is ten times as toxic as lead, and its effects are ten times more damaging. Cadmium was not found above the earth's crust prior to industrialization. Now it can be detected almost everywhere. Cadmium enters the body through air, water, and food sources, and can attack every system of the body.

It is stored in the tissues of the human body, mostly in the kidneys and the liver. Its half-life in the body is approximately 10 to 25 years, so whatever amount of cadmium you have in your body at any given time, you will still have half of that amount in your body 10 to 25 years later.

Any amount of cadmium will cause irreparable damage to body cells. Its main toxic effects are exerted on the heart, liver, and kidneys. It also affects the brain and other cells of the nervous system. Cadmium is extremely neurotoxic — excesses can be lethal.

Acute cadmium toxicity usually occurs in job settings. Welders, for example, are regularly exposed to cadmium. There is usually a delay of several hours before the initial effects of acute cadmium poisoning are noticeable. These first effects include nausea and vomiting. As time progresses, degeneration of body tissues becomes evident. The chronic degenerative effects of cadmium poisoning are exceptionally devastating. Cadmium will attack and destroy any body tissue that it is housed in. Cadmium is known to destroy lung tissue, and has been linked with some cases of asthma and bronchitis. It causes excessive damage to the nervous tissue of the brain and spinal cord. It can cause gangrene in the testicles. It is also linked to testicular cancer and some skin cancers. Chronic cadmium toxicity will cause anemia. There is also a strong association with kidney disease. Cadmium can cause delicate kidney tissues to slough off and be excreted in the urine in severe cases of chronic toxicity. Excessive cadmium generally concentrates in the kidneys. As it concentrates it causes damage which initially shows up as hypertension (high blood pressure). Once cadmium is removed, blood pressure can generally be restored to reasonable levels if kidney function has not been irreparably damaged. Cadmium has also been implicated in bone disease, cancerous tissues, and emphysema. Cadmium has many other negative effects: it causes a decrease in hydroxylation or conversion of vitamin D from inactive to active form (as described on page 58), is associated with a five-fold increase in hypertension, can cause kidney and liver failure, lung failure, hardening of the arteries, and decreased myocardial or heart function, is associated with anemia, pregnancy toxemia, and testicular necrosis, and is commonly found at increased levels in patients with prostate cancer. Cadmium has a teratogenic effect on pregnancy — it causes birth defects — and is mutagenic — it causes genetic defects. The presence of cadmium has been shown to decrease verbal intelligence quotient scores and it has been found in higher concentrations where children have either been dyslexic or have had borderline retardation. As you can see, cadmium presents a huge health hazard to human life, both in children and adults. It is extremely toxic.

Most cadmium is ingested from food but some comes from air and smoke. The smallest amount is absorbed from water. The acceptable level of cadmium in the soil is 1 part per million. Fourteen percent of Canadian communities are above this level. Soil in mining cities such as Flin Flon, Manitoba, contains between 50 and 350 parts per million. Tuktoyaktuk in the Northwest Territories contains 55 parts per million. North American codfish contains 11 parts per million and oysters contain on the average 56 parts per million. The health effects of cadmium are similar to those of lead. When both metals are present in the body, cadmium potentiates the toxic effects of lead in a synergistic or multiplier effect rather than in an additive effect — that is, lead and cadmium together are many times more toxic than lead or cadmium alone.

This synergistic effect was demonstrated in an experiment published in the *Journal of Toxicology and Environmental Health* in 1978. The authors, J. Schubert, E.J. Riley, and S.A. Tyler, demonstrated that the combination of any two of cadmium, mercury, and lead was dramatically more toxic where the most toxic metal was present in a dosage high enough to produce a death in 1 out of 100 tested rats. Introduction of a smaller amount of a less toxic metal produced a much higher than expected death rate. This phenomenon may have significant clinical application where a patient has severe symptoms of neurological compromise with detectable levels of two or more toxic heavy metals.

Humans are not ordinarily born with cadmium in their body tissues, although our environment and our mothers are sometimes so toxic that placental transfer must be considered a source of toxicity. Cadmium can pass through the placenta into the developing fetus, although there is a naturally occurring metal-binding protein which is secreted by the placenta called metallothionein which offers some protection. It binds to cadmium molecules and blocks their transfer through the placenta unless there is so much cadmium that it overwhelms this protein. Excess cadmium then crosses the placenta freely.

Research has shown that cadmium is commonly seen in

developing infants once breastfeeding is initiated. Cadmium does appear in breastmilk

Cadmium today is used largely in electroplating iron and steel. It is durable and protects and improves the appearance of metal wares. It is used in industrial equipment, screws, nuts, bolts, and other miscellaneous hardware items, and can be found in galvanized products such as nails, pipes, and fluid containers. There have been situations where carpenters became toxic from holding metal nails in their mouths. Wines prepared and stored in galvanized containers have also caused problems. Cadmium is used in automobile parts and electrical and electronic products. It is a metal of choice for such wares as it has excellent anti-corrosive properties. It has also been used as an automotive lubricant and it is emitted in car exhaust, probably after it is picked up from automotive parts and lubricants.

Cadmium has been used as pigment for paint since the 1930s. It provides excellent yellow, orange, red, and maroon pigments which are extremely durable and long-lasting. It is found in glazes, too, particularly those which have a bright yellow or red color. Acidic foods or fluids will leach cadmium out of glazes.

Cadmium is found in PVC piping, and can leach out of the plastic pipes. It is also present in copper pipes and can leach out of them as well, especially if your water tends to be acidic.

Cadmium has long been used for solder. This puts welders at high risk for cadmium toxicity as a job hazard.

It is a common component of many batteries. Used in a combination with nickel (nicad batteries), cadmium helps to pick up and hold a charge longer than many other metals. Nicad batteries are commonly used as rechargeable batteries today, posing a risk if the battery's structure is damaged as it will then leak toxic material. There is also a question of how and where these batteries will be discarded.

A cigarette can contain 1 to 2 µg of cadmium per cigarette. A smoker's intake of cadmium is twice that of a non smoker. Cadmium is also found in shoe polish, fungicides, in the photographic and engraving industry, in semi-conductors and in rubber tires (it is a major contaminant of the environment in this form, as rubber tires are discarded and break down).

Mercury

Mercury is another poison that appears in our environment more than we would like to acknowledge. First of all, 30,000 to 150,000 tons are released into the atmosphere annually through a natural process called "degassing." This is the natural emission of mercury from Earth's crust in vapor form. It is also emitted through volcanic activity. Combustion of fossil fuels releases 5000 tons per year into the atmosphere, and 15,000 tons are mined annually throughout the world. A long list of uses will follow but who can provide one example where mercury ends up being reclaimed? Most of it ends up dissipating into our environment.

Mercury has long been known to cause deterioration of the nervous system. During the nineteenth century, manufacturers of felt hats used mercuric nitrate as a tanning solution for the felt. Following prolonged exposure to and inhalation of the fumes, these hat makers developed symptoms of tremor, fatigue, headache, excitability, and, in later stages, behavior and personality changes, memory loss, and psychosis consisting of delirium and hallucinations. Hence the origin of the phrase "mad as a hatter." Unfortunately, no treatment was known that would remove the mercury.

In the 1960s, 500 people died in the Minamata Bay area of Japan when they developed mercury poisoning after eating contaminated seafood caught in the bay. The seafood was contaminated by a mercury-containing catalyst that was dumped into the bay by a local factory producing chlorine bleach. While hair mercury levels of 5 parts per million are deemed to be toxic, Minamata residents had levels of 183 parts per million.

Another similar catastrophe, known as the Ramadan flour disaster, occurred in Iraq in both 1956 and 1960. Grain seed which had been provided for sowing had been treated with a mercury-containing fungicide with the assumption that all of the seed would end up being planted. Unfortunately, much of the seed was ground into flour and used for baking. Some was also used as feed for chickens, which caused the meat to become contaminated. As a result, 459 people died and 6530 were admitted to hospitals. Hair sample analysis showed mercury levels higher than 500 parts per million. In 1966, Guatemala had the same type of problem with mercury-treated seeds, and in 1969, in Alberta, Canada, excessive mercury was found in wild pheasant and the province had to shut down that year's hunting season.

The consequences of acute mercury poisoning are terrible. The actual toxic effect takes approximately one to three months to become obvious, but in that time mercury demolishes the nerve cells of the brain and destroys granular cells in the cerebellum. In extreme cases of mercury poisoning, the initial onset is signalled by visual problems. This soon leads to blindness, after which extreme dementia occurs. People may become so brain-damaged that they run around screaming, falling, jumping out of windows, completely oblivious to this world. There have been cases of severe mercury poisoning where patients have had to be put in strait jackets to protect them. During the mercury poisoning incidents in Japan and Iraq, hospital wards were filled with screaming, moaning, incontinent humans who had to be restrained as they awaited death. Mercifully, coma and death do follow severe mercury poisoning.

As mercury causes subtle effects which are typically not recognized at low concentrations, symptoms of chronic mercury toxicity are hard to detect. Many recent studies indicate a direct relationship to changes in mental health. Symptoms include irritability, excitability, outbursts of temper, extreme shyness and avoidance of strangers, anxiety, tension, depression, fatigue, and forgetfulness. Some of the more severe symptoms are hallucinations, suicidal tendencies, melancholia, and manic-depressive psychosis.

Some of the characteristics of chronic mercury poisoning are slowed motor and mental functions analogous to Parkinsonism, dementia similar to Alzheimer's disease with memory loss and behavioral changes, peripheral nerve damage resulting in uncoordinated gait, restriction of visual fields, hearing loss, depression and weakness. Mercury can cause difficulty with chewing and swallowing, and involuntary muscle movement. Toxicity may initially show up as dizziness. Severe mercury poisoning can lead to a loss of control of limbs or impaired vision (often leading to blindness), and it has been suspected as the cause in some cases of multiple sclerosis. At lower levels, decreased concentration and difficulty with learning may be the only symptoms.

There are now studies which indicate a direct correlation between mercury and behavior problems, learning problems, a decrease in verbal IQ , and reduced academic ability at levels below those known to cause the classical symptoms of mercury toxicity. Rats that were exposed to low levels of mercury vapor were found to have increased spontaneous aggressive behavior. Anger is a common symptom of mercury toxicity.

In a study conducted in Russia on newborn babies that were exposed to mercury *in utero*, seven out of ten babies were found to be mentally retarded. Mercury has a strong affinity for brain tissue. Its neurotoxic results are devastating.

Mercury is mutagenic. Chromosomal changes can show up in offspring many generations down the line as a result of acute and/or chronic mercury poisoning.

Mercury can be found in the air as mercury vapor and is

released into the air when coal is burned. It is another element that has been added to household paints for many decades. It can be found in water. It is sometimes present in the food we eat.

Perhaps one of the most controversial areas of mercury usage is in the field of dentistry where mercury makes up 50 percent of an amalgam filling. Mercury has been banned for this use in Germany and in parts of Scandinavia. Dentists and other personnel working in the dental field as well as their families are at significant risk. Many recent studies have been conducted relating dental amalgams to the silent, chronic effects of mercury toxicity and the psychological disorders that it imposes. Research clearly shows that, over a long period of time, small amounts of mercury exposure can produce the same devastating effects as excessive exposure in a short time period. As 80 percent of the world's dental cavities are filled with dental amalgam (silver fillings which are 50 percent mercury), many people are susceptible to the effects of this metal. Silver fillings are an unstable alloy; they continuously release elemental mercury. The amount of released mercury when measured can be directly related to the number of dental amalgams. J. Pleva, a corrosion scientist in Sweden, revealed that five-year-old dental amalgam had lost half of its mercury from the chewing surface. He also found that after twenty years, the amalgam had no mercury left on the chewing surface. It was after he discovered the corrosion of his own dental amalgams that he began to suspect that he, himself, was suffering from chronic mercury toxicity. He found that within three months of having his amalgams removed, his symptoms of anxiety, irritability, indecision, tiredness, feeling stressed, and resistance to intellectual work had disappeared.

Mercury is released from dental amalgams in the form of mercury vapor which is inhaled into the lungs and then absorbed into the blood. Once in the bloodstream it passes through the blood-brain barrier and becomes sequestered in the brain tissue as organic methyl mercury. To date there have been many studies indicating a direct correlation between the number of silver dental amalgams in a person's teeth and mercury concentration in the brain.

By far the most common use of mercury is in the electrical and chloralkali industries. The chloralkali industry uses mercury as a catalyst to produce chlorine bleaching agents for the pulp and paper industry. There has been a gradual shift to using hydrogen peroxide, but large areas have been contaminated and are still being contaminated by pulp mills using chlorine to bleach pulp. Rivers, streams, lakes, and some coastal areas are common receptacles for these contaminated effluents.

Mercury is commonly used in the paint industry. Fifteen percent of all mined mercury ends up as an anti-foulant in paints. Measurable amounts of mercury are emitted from interior latex paints at the rate of approximately 500 nanomoles per day for as long as seven and a half years. In addition to that, EPA standards of 1.5 millimoles of mercury per litre of paint are frequently exceeded. Levels as much as 1000 percent above the EPA limits have been found during investigations. Another 10 percent of mined mercury is used in the surgical instrument industry, 5 percent is used as a fungicide in seed grains, and 3 percent is used in wood fungicides and slug killers.

Mercury is still found in some fungal medicines, lotions, eyedrops, and cosmetics. Mercury also finds its way into batteries, vapor lamps, polishes, and household cleaners as well as detonators for explosives. The leather tanning industry still uses mercury. Mercury is commonly found in seafoods. The larger the fish, the more likelihood of mercury contamination. The usual amount of mercury in uncontaminated seafoods is approximately 1 µg/kg. In Minamata Bay, levels in fish reached 11 µg/kg and some shellfish had 36 µg/kg. There have been cases of children exposed to the contents of a broken mercury thermometer developing signs of mercury poisoning. The amount of mercury that is released into our environment and never accounted for again is appalling.

Arsenic

In nature arsenic is distributed throughout the earth's crust. It appears in varying amounts in most water supplies and is incorporated into plants. Although it has no known function in the human body, research suggests that a very small amount of arsenic is acceptable (perhaps even required) in the human body, and a certain level is expected to be seen in a laboratory sample of human tissue and body fluids. Current research also indicates that it is frequently found in body tissues in amounts that exceed the acceptable levels.

The main toxic effects of elevated levels of arsenic are extreme fatigue, energy loss, inflammation of the stomach and intestines, kidney degeneration, cirrhosis of the liver, bone marrow degeneration, and nervous system damage. It has been linked to some forms of cancer and has been demonstrated to cause skin and lung cancers in test animals.

Arsenic causes many other adverse health effects including acceleration of atherosclerosis, hair loss, sensory and motor nerve damage, and decrease in cognitive function. Specifically, tasks involving word use and spelling seem to be noticeably affected. Arsenicals can paralyze smooth muscle (those muscles which produce slow long-term contractions, like the ones in the hollow organs such as stomach, intestine, blood vessels, and bladder), and can cause pain and discomfort in the extremities. Arsenic blocks a process known as oxidative phosphorylation — a process by which oxygen-breathing organisms, including humans, produce energy in the form of a high-energy phosphate bond.

When lead and arsenic co-exist in a child's body, the combination of the two has been found to have a synergistic effect. Researchers have documented that the combined negative effect exceeds the sum of their independent effects.

Fifty thousand tons of arsenic are produced annually in the United States. Thirty thousand tons are used to make insecticides, pesticides, herbicides, rodenticides, and fungicides. It is also used as a wood preservative and as an antifoulant in paint. It is added to lubricating oils, can be found in ceramics and glass, and is also a product of coal burning. Feed additives may contain arsenic to control gastric pathogens, particularly in pigs and poultry. Arsenic is occasionally found in unusually high levels in drinking water, and its presence is a fairly common problem in well water in some areas. Seafoods have an especially high content of arsenic.

One of the most toxic gases is arsene, the gaseous form of arsenic. Concentrations of 250 parts per million in air can be lethal in 30 minutes. Arsene is produced in the smelting and refining of arsenic-containing scrap metal and in the initial smelting of copper, lead, and zinc-bearing ores which often contain high levels of arsenic.

Nickel

Nickel, one of the most common elements in the earth's crust, is thought to occur in large quantities in the earth's core, and appears in trace amounts in seawater. It appears in some kinds of meteorites.

Elevated levels of nickel have been known to cause disorders of the central nervous system, stomach, and intestines. It can cause an excess in blood sugar and has been shown to cause heart, brain, liver, and kidney disorders in animals.

Nickel is used largely in the stainless steel industry. It is also used in coins, ceramics, special chemical-containing vessels, rechargeable batteries, electronic circuits, and dyes.

Aluminum

Aluminum is the most abundant metallic element on both Earth and the moon. It is found in various mineral complexes, primarily bauxite, and makes up 8 percent of Earth's surface. It can be found widely distributed in plant life. Almost all rocks contain some aluminum.

Current evidence indicates that aluminum in large quantities causes damage to the nervous system. It too has a synergistic toxic effect when it is present in the body with lead. It can be responsible for brain disorders, has a well known link to dementia and some forms of epilepsy, and has recently received considerable attention due to increased levels found in Alzheimer patients.

Aluminum has been shown to interfere with memory and cognitive function and has also been identified as an ophthalmic, or eye motor nerve, paralytic agent. Elevated aluminum in humans has been associated with depressed visual motor performance. Increased hair aluminum has been associated with decreased upper limb coordination and visual motor/fine motor control. (These types of disruptions in children have been considered as early signs of brain damage.) In studies of some institutionalized boys displaying psychotic or prepsychotic behaviors, hair aluminum was found to be seven times more prevalent than in typical patients. There is a strong suggestion that chronic aluminum toxicity can be a causative factor in childhood hyperactivity, psychosis, and congenital anomalies.

Aluminum can bind to iron-binding sites in hemoglobin, displacing iron and causing microcytic or small-cell anemia. It readily crosses the blood-brain barrier where it interferes with several enzyme systems. By binding to acetyl choline transferase, it can decrease the production of acetyl choline, a nerve transmitter substance. It can block beta dopamine hydroxylase and thereby decrease the production of dopamine, a neurotransmitter which is also a precursor to adrenalin. Perhaps the reason why some children who are metal toxic respond to Ritalin is because they have a generalized dopamine deficiency, and the Ritalin — an adrenalin-like substance — provides that missing link.

High levels of aluminum have been associated not only

with neurological dysfunction but also with damage to the kidneys and heart. The metal can interfere with enzymes which eliminate or neutralize ammonia, a poisonous waste product, in the body. It can cross the placenta and cause not only the above noted problems but also a generalized impairment of infant growth and development.

Foods can pick up this metal when they are cooked and stored in aluminum containers. Think of all the food containers, wrappers, foils, etc. that allow direct contact of food or drink items with aluminum. It is found as a drying agent in various foods including baking soda, coffee whitener, and table salt, is applied to the skin as an anti-perspirant, and is frequently found in treated drinking water. Other common sources of aluminum include antacids, salt, and pop cans. Interestingly, the aluminum content in soft drinks can be as high as 30 micromoles per litre. Beer, on the other hand, is estimated to contain an average of 6 micromoles per litre. For all the beer lovers, this may come as good news.

Soil in areas of high volcanic activity is particularly contaminated. People living near smelters or working in the welding and fabricating industry are susceptible to aluminum exposure and should use proper protection.

Young children may be exposed to aluminum when they are vaccinated. Vaccines can contain aluminum, thimerosal (a preservative which contains mercury), formaldehyde, and various animal proteins that are used to weaken or attenuate the vaccine. Aluminum is used as an "adjuvant," to speed up the body's antibody or immune response to the vaccine antigen. The vaccine, which is supposed to trigger an immune response that will train the immune system to produce antibodies coded to destroy the foreign organisms with which the child is inoculated, could theoretically be causing an auto-immune response. Because aluminum tends to accumulate in neurological tissues, the child's body might be destroying its own nervous system in its effort to eliminate the foreign metal-protein complex. This may be a key as to why some children show more sensitivity to various metals than other children do.

Tin

Tin, which has been used for at least 4000 years, is also not good stuff. It is extremely toxic and can cause neurological deficits such as depression, encephalopathy, cerebral edema, and in some cases headache, seizure, and coma. It can also be inhaled and causes a lung disease called pneumoconiosis. Tin is a powerful immunosuppressant.

When it's alloyed with other metals tin is not as toxic unless it comes in contact with acidic juices such as tomato juice for prolonged periods of time. Food cans are still made of tin, and it is also used in the ceramic and textile industry.

Tin alloys readily with copper to produce bronze. It is used largely in electroplating and is frequently used to coat steel containers that are then used for many different types of foods and beverages. It is also used as a catalyst in rubber production, a stabilizer in PVC resins, an anti-foulant in paint, a sanitizing agent, and a wood preservative. It is commonly used in eating utensils and in roofing materials.

ESSENTIAL TRACE ELEMENTS

It is thought that heavy metals produce many of their toxic effects by displacing essential trace minerals. Doctors and parents must therefore be aware that some trace mineral deficiencies can also be contributing to neurological dysfunction. Low levels of lithium, for example, have been identified in one Texas community with an increased incidence of antisocial and criminal behavior. We have seen several cases where children with low levels of lithium and the symptoms of hyperactivity have improved with the administration of small amounts of lithium carbonate.

We will only mention the essential elements that are

known to pose a serious health threat to young children when in decreased or toxic quantities in a human body. This is not to say that all individuals with these toxicities will demonstrate all of the known effects — some clearly do not exhibit all or any of them. As with any health problem there is individual variability whereby some bodies are more sensitive than others and have more symptoms than others even with similar quantities of toxic elements.

Copper

Copper, the twentieth most common element present in the earth's crust, often appears in its pure form in nature and is an essential element in the human body. Certain amounts are necessary for adequate enzyme function. However, excessive amounts can have extremely devastating effects on the human body, particularly that of the developing child.

Ingestion of large quantities of copper can cause irritation of the stomach and intestines. Excessive absorption of copper can produce toxic effects such as anemia, loss of hair pigment, reduced growth, and loss of arterial wall elasticity. It can also cause cirrhosis of the liver and other liver diseases. Copper can be fatal at high doses.

Excess copper stored in the liver, brain, and corneal cells has long been associated with Wilson's disease, a devastating disease where degenerative changes in the brain nerve cells become evident as mental retardation and symptoms resembling Parkinsonism. If this disease is properly detected and diagnosed it is possible to prevent further liver and brain damage by treatment with chelating agents. Cuprimine is one agent proven to be extremely effective in the treatment of Wilson's disease.

Copper alone can be the cause of severe neurological impairment in a child. One summary of 51 studies involving young children found an association between excessive hair copper and undesirable behavior. In another study, hair copper levels in dyslexic children were found to be nearly double those of the control group (although the levels of copper from both groups were reported to be within the acceptable range). The presence of elevated copper along with other metals in excess is thought to be significant.

Copper has recently been identified as a contributing factor to atherosclerotic disease. It causes increased levels of low-density lipoprotein to accumulate in the inner blood vessel walls and attack cell membranes. High storage levels are associated with excess risk of myocardial infarction or heart attack. It has also been found to adversely affect mental function and development.

Chromium

Chromium is a non-corrosive, high-strength, heat-resistant metal that rarely occurs in nature. It is vital to glucose metabolism, fat metabolism, heart functions, and other important metabolic functions. A lack of chromium increases the toxic effects of lead.

Chromium deficiencies are generally more common than excesses. Chromium deficiency mimics diabetes mellitus, a disorder of carbohydrate metabolism in which body sugars are not oxidized to produce energy due to lack of the pancreatic hormone insulin, or to resistance to insulin. Some studies have shown hair chromium to be significantly depressed in patients with juvenile onset diabetes as well as adults with diabetes. Incidentally, hair chromium decreases with age. So does glucose tolerance.

Chromium is used mostly for electroplating coatings and in stainless steel production. It is also used in enamels, as an addition to cast iron, and in wire.

Molybdenum

The name molybdenum is derived from the Greek word "molybdos," meaning "lead-like." It was discovered in 1778 by K.W. Scheele but was not used industrially until World War I at which time the Germans used molybdenum or "moly steel" in their "Big Bertha" gun barrels. Molybdenum can be found in many parts of the world, but the richest deposits are in the western hemisphere. Two thirds to three quarters of the world's output comes from mining operations and the remainder is recovered as a by-product of copper mining.

Molybdenum is another trace element that may or may not belong in the essential elements group. At elevated levels this element causes irritation of the eyes, nose, and throat. It can also cause gout and bone disorders, loss of appetite, anemia, loss of hair and hair color, and bone defects.

Molybdenum is used in electronic devices, contacts, electrodes, transducers, and transistors. It is also used in the die-casting of aluminum and as an automotive lubricant.

Silver

Silver is a rather rare heavy metal which sometimes appears as a free element in nature.

High levels of silver are neurotoxic. They are known to cause central nervous system disorders.

Zinc

The discovery of zinc is prehistoric. It is found in ores, in seawater, and in virtually every type of human food as it is readily absorbed from the soil. Zinc usually co-occurs with lead in its natural form.

Zinc is an essential element, necessary in almost every biochemical system of the human body. It appears in a wide variety of biological compounds: proteins, amino acids, nucleic acids, and porphyrins. It helps the body to maintain healthy cells and is necessary for growth. Acceptable levels of zinc are known to protect the body from the effects of lead and cadmium.

Some of the more common effects of excessive zinc include irritation, stiffness, muscle pain, a decrease in appetite, and nausea. Zinc toxicity has been known to inhibit growth. Absence of zinc can cause loss of taste, loss of appetite, and a decrease in fertility. Deficiency is also associated with prostatic hypertrophy in adult men.

Iron

Iron is the fourth most abundant metal found in Earth's crust, accounting for 5 percent of the metals in the crust. It is found naturally occurring with many other minerals and in ground water. It is believed that iron was first extracted from ore around 3000 BC.

Excessive iron can cause gastro-intestinal irritation and necrosis, hematemesis, lethargy, hypotension, coma, pulmonary edema, respiratory failure, and death. High levels of iron have recently been identified as a risk factor in atherosclerotic heart disease.

An association between depressed iron levels and anemia has long been recognized. Now it is also recognized that when both copper and iron are depressed, anemia is often observed.

By far the most common use of iron today is in steel production. Steel is a generic name for a large group of iron alloys, so it appears in most steel structures. It is used to make cast iron and wrought iron. It also is used in magnets, dyes, abrasives, and in magnetic circuits.

Manganese

Manganese is the twelfth most abundant element in Earth's crust. In proper amounts, manganese, like other trace minerals, is essential in activating enzymes, particularly those which break down proteins and those which are necessary for energy production in the body. In excess, manganese causes serious toxic symptoms. It has been associated with chronic fatigue, diffuse muscle and joint pains, disorders of coordination and movement, speech disorders, Parkinson-like symptoms of masked facies (no facial expression), tremor, slow movement, slow speech, and a slowing of thought processes.

Many studies involving hair manganese and children's behavior have revealed a tendency for lowered hair manganese in learning-disabled children and in juvenile delinquents. There have also been associations made between depressed hair manganese and allergies, joint problems, and congenital abnormalities. Chronic manganism (low manganese) is uncommon but when it does occur the first clinical signs are typically disrupted mental processes. When patients exhibiting manganism are given manganese supplements, improvements are generally seen.

In some studies hair manganese has been found to be lower in schizophrenic patients than in other patients. It has also been shown to be significantly reduced in multiple sclerosis patients.

Manganese has recently been substituted for lead as an anti-knocking compound in gasoline. Although the use of manganese has been decreased because it plugs catalytic convertors in cars, the metal can still be found in jet fuels.

Manganese is also used in dry cell batteries, ceramics and glass dyes, as a hardener of steel alloys, and in the manufacture of matches, paints, and pesticides.

Although there are many other essential and non-essential trace elements and metals we have not mentioned that are found in body tissues, the health hazards posed by them are not clear.

Another significant piece of information to bear in mind is that, hand-in-hand with lead and other heavy metal toxicities comes the additional problem of nutritional deficiencies. There is a strong link between nutritional deficiencies and metal toxicity, although the actual chemistry of the combination is not completely clear. Children with lead and other metal toxicities almost always have trace element deficiencies, diet problems, and in some instances weight loss and pica. The fact that toxic metals are known to displace essential trace minerals is one issue, the gut problems caused by intestinal irritation leading to a lack of appetite (and therefore inadequate nutrition) is another. Along with this comes inadequate trace mineral intake to keep enzymes functioning to maintain normal body functioning. Where trace mineral intake is deficient, there is further malabsorption. This creates a vicious circle.

In the case of my children, Cam and Brett were extremely deficient in lithium, vanadium, strontium, and silicon. They had an over-abundance of copper, cadmium, tin, aluminum, manganese, chromium, phosphorous, arsenic, and, of course, lead. In elevated quantities, these elements are all harmful to children. Having neurological damage from toxic metals is one huge insult, but consider this neurological insult in combination with the nutritional or trace element deficiencies. For one example, lithium is directly related to optimal mental functioning, but it is frequently deficient in kids with high levels of lead. What a sad combination for neurological damage.

One frequently asked question is "Why is this a problem now?" Some of these metals have been around for centuries, and all have been used in large quantities throughout the twentieth century — how come children are just suffering developmental problems now? Well, we don't know how many children were affected before without being diagnosed as metal toxic. As a result of improved testing techniques over the last few decades, we have been made more aware of how pervasive and long-standing this problem is. But today's children are facing not only ever-increasing industrialization and resulting pollution, but also the metals that have been brought above the earth's surface over the past centuries — metals that don't break down or go away.

Five billion pounds of chemicals are brought into the environment per year. This is equivalent to 25 pounds for each square mile of earth surface annually. In the United States alone it is estimated that 6 million tons of aluminum waste and 126,000 tons of lead in various wasted forms enter into the North American environment annually.

Ice samples taken in Greenland and compared to samples deeper down, at approximately the 800 BC level, show that there has been a 200-fold increase in lead in the environment, with two peaks occurring during the industrial revolution and upon the introduction of leaded gasoline in 1920. The body burden of lead in industrialized modern man is said to be between 500 and 1400 times higher than in individuals living in primitive societies.

As the world becomes more industrialized, nature is becoming more compromised. The air is contaminated throughout the world, particularly in the northern hemisphere where most industrialized development has occurred. Millions of tons of gaseous waste and other toxic particles rise into the atmosphere and are distributed around the globe. Mountain ranges form basins which collect the precipitants as they drop from the skies in solution — what we know as acid rain. Water is not only acidified, it is also contaminated with metal particles and other toxins. As air masses, in the form of shifting wind currents, readily distribute metal-laden moisture from one part of the globe to another, we can see that the effort to decrease atmospheric lead and other heavy metals must be an international one.

Industry also releases massive tonnages of industrial waste into river systems which slowly poison the food chain from plants and fish to man. It is estimated that the Mississippi River is a toxic dump for 2000 tons of cadmium annually. Cadmium, more toxic than lead, is just one item of the many that are dumped into that river system.

The acid water that either comes down as rain or floats down our rivers is corrosive. As the water is treated for humans, pH levels stay on the low (acidic) side, and when the water passes through our pipes it leaches heavy metals into solution. In some older cities it was common, around the turn of the century, to follow the example of the Romans and to use solid lead piping for some of the larger water mains. Some oldtimers tell stories about lead pipes being used in homes in decades gone by.

Copper piping has also become a hazard, particularly where pH levels in water have dropped. To add to the problem, copper pipes are not pure copper. Residual amounts of zinc, cadmium, and lead remain in trace amounts following the smelting process. Soldered joints in older homes still contain as much as 50 percent lead. Solders are now being made of other metallic materials but there are no guarantees that these are any less toxic than the lead was.

Through water, air, and soil contamination, these different toxins end up in the food chain. Plants absorb and incorporate heavy metals into their biochemical systems in the same way that humans do. In fact, plants have been used by some environmental experts to extract heavy metals from contaminated soils. Once plants used for this purpose are saturated with these toxic metals, they are harvested and dumped somewhere else. Unfortunately, the same extraction processes occur in our edible plants and these are disposed of on our dining room tables.

And to counter questions about why this is only happening now, there have been dramatic examples of metal poisoning in the past. We've already mentioned how metals may have contributed to the fall of the Roman Empire and the madness of nineteenth century hatmakers. Historians believe lead poisoning may have contributed to the fate of the John Franklin expedition in 1845. One hundred thirty-three men perished over a period of two years as they tried to find their way through the Northwest Passage. Diaries describe increasingly bizarre behavior on the part of the lost explorers. They made a ridiculous attempt to drag massive amounts of material, including a lifeboat, across 1000 kilometres of barren ice. Only their diaries survived to tell the story. When the bodies of expedition members were exhumed, scientists were able to determine that body tissues contained poisonous levels of lead. This could be accounted for by the lead-soldered cans containing their foodstuffs.

All historical poisonings have not been unintentional. When hair analysis was performed upon Napoleon, it was determined that toxic levels of arsenic were present, though there is debate over the significance of this discovery.

More recently, major epidemics of lead poisoning broke out following both World War II and the Korean war. Military personnel used large quantities of lead-based paints as an anti-corrosive on ships and land-based war machinery. Based on the medical community's experiences treating these war veterans, modern techniques of detoxification were developed.

Consciously or unconsciously, we've been poisoning ourselves for centuries and as you are now well aware, the stuff is everywhere.

10

Prevention

Completely avoiding exposure to lead and other metals is impossible in any industrialized city. Avoiding excessive exposure is not. Once you start to become aware of the sources described in previous chapters, you will soon develop a sense of where you will find them in your daily environment. You will also be able to develop some strategies for reducing your family's risk of exposure, particularly where pregnant women and young children are involved.

Paint and renovations

The number one source of childhood lead poisoning remains household paint. Despite the 1978 ban on leaded paint, old lead-based paints still are estimated to cover the walls of approximately 54 million homes in the United States alone. If your home was built before 1978 you will likely have lead-based paint on both exterior and interior surfaces. This is perhaps the most common avenue of exposure for both chronic and acute cases of lead toxicity.

About 75 percent of all houses in the United States built before 1980 contain lead paint and some newer homes are also contaminated. It is estimated that there are approximately 1.3 million tons of lead paint in American housing. The Alliance to End Childhood Lead Poisoning estimates that almost 4 million houses and apartments in the U.S. have chipping and peeling lead paint producing hazardous levels of lead dust exposure for the inhabitants. In 1992 the Centers for Disease Control estimated that 12 million American children under seven years of age were exposed to lead paint. During the 1950s there was a noticeable increase in childhood lead poisoning. Leaded house paint from the previous half century of housing was cited as the culprit. By 1953 the paint industry voluntarily issued standards limiting lead to account for only 1 percent of all the additives in house paint. In 1971 the United States Congress passed the Lead Paint Poisoning Act which prohibited the use of lead-based paints on surfaces which were accessible to children. Congress also set up grant programs that paid for screening and treatment of children suspected of lead-paint exposure. By 1973 Congress amended the act to prohibit the use of paint containing more than .5 percent lead in federally funded housing. This act also applied to paint for toys and other sources which children might be exposed to. Most paint sold before 1970 contained excessive lead. If your house was built before 1950 there is a high probability that much of the paint contains high levels of lead. Any chipping or peeling paint will pose an immediate health threat to fetuses and children. It would be safe to assume that it will also pose a serious health threat to adults.

Lead was used as a pigment in many paints shortly after World War II, particularly in white and pastel shades. These paints often contained as much as 50 percent lead (by weight). In the 1950s, some other pigments were used to replace lead, however smaller amounts of lead were still used in some paints and sealants. Many of these lead-based paints were sold in more recent years as trim paints, commonly used around window and door frames. Many paints developed for metal coverage — for bridges, children's toys and furniture, etc. — contained large amounts of lead. Some paints also contain cadmium, mercury, and other metals.

Currently the Hazardous Products Act prohibits lead from being used in paint in the U.S. However the problem still exists in many homes, particularly those that are over 40 years old. Many compounds of lead are used in the manufacture of household building materials (sheathing for telephone and cable wires, PVC pipes and other plastics, glass, roofing, flashings, etc.). These can expose occupants of affected homes to serious health hazards.

Take this information and give some thought to the dangers presented when these older homes (and some not even all that old) are renovated. This is another huge opportunity for exposure to lead and other heavy metals. I can't help but reflect on all of the minor and some not-so-minor renovations that my husband and I carried out on our home. Our first house, built in the 1970s, had a basement suite built and plumbed in after we bought it. We had new plumbing fixtures put in after the children were born. It also had another previously unfinished basement room completed. We had two large decks built, a few inside walls opened up and removed, a wood-burning fireplace installed, and the floor coverings replaced. In the process there was exposure to every type of product used in the housing industry. Walls, paint, flooring, etc. were sanded, scraped, cut, and removed with no concern for the particles of dust and debris that these processes create. We were not the least bit aware of the hazards that we were exposed to in our daily activities at that point. I recall the children and I were often an audience for the workers doing the renovations. We loved to sit and watch what was going on. If I had only known!

I look at the backgrounds of many of the children who are now testing positive for long-term body burden of metals, and many of them have been exposed to major house renovations. I suppose that parents of my generation have been buying the older houses as they are more affordable and then, as we achieve financial stability, we renovate them to meet our families' needs. Little do we realize we are creating a huge health hazard for our developing fetuses and children. We are also poisoning ourselves.

Hazardous amounts of lead dust can be created by something as simple as opening and shutting a window or door that has been painted with a lead-based paint. As these dust particles fall to the floor, our children, particularly infants and toddlers, are crawling right through them. They are breathing the dust, they are picking up the particles on their hands, feet, clothing, and toys. Because of the constant hand to mouth activity in their early years, toddlers end up ingesting the lead dust and, as we now know, their bodies are absorbing this lead and storing it in their body tissues. We are not even talking about renovation exposure at this stage. This is everyday exposure for a child in an older, lead-painted home.

As children start to play outside the home they become exposed to more lead dust, chips, particles, etc. that are in the exterior house paint. These particles fall to the ground and remain in the soil. They do not go away. Lead just doesn't disappear. It continues to accumulate over the years and contaminates the soil. Young children are exposed as they crawl around their yards, play with their toys, test out new rocks and shrubs for flavor and texture, etc.

With this knowledge it is important to start to look for potential lead and other metal hazards in your home. It is especially important if your house is very old, but don't be fooled into feeling comfortable if your house is not a relic. Metals can still be a problem.

If you live in an older home and you know or suspect that it contains lead-based paint, don't panic and sell. Paint is not harmful if it is in good condition. You will have to look carefully for flaking or chipping areas of paint. The dust from the crumbling old particles of paint must be carefully removed and disposed of as it will inevitably end up in your home, your soil, and/or your child's body. It might contaminate your garden and could end up in the food that you grow and prepare for your family. Or it may end up in your child's play area or sandbox.

If you are not sure if your home contains lead-based paint you can easily have paint chips tested by a lab. There is also a test kit that can be purchased and used by the consumer that will detect lead in paint. The most important requirement, though, should be careful monitoring and eventual covering up or removal of such areas of your home that might contain lead or other metals. Remember that renovations and removal of lead-affected materials will be hazardous to humans and animals. Lead paint can be professionally removed by qualified technicians and disposed of in a safe manner. Leaded areas can also be treated with a strong phosphate solution (such as trisodium phosphate, or TSP) and then covered up permanently with a layer of lead-free paint, paneling, siding, etc. This is only recommended if the leaded area is in relatively good shape.

It is essential to protect yourself while working with contaminated areas as you will be exposed to the lead. Strict precautions should always be taken when removing leaded materials from your home. Window sills, baseboards, doors, mouldings, etc. can be removed and replaced with unleaded ones, but you must be extremely careful not to disturb the paint when removing these items. You can contact your municipal waste management agency or the ministry of the environment to find out how to dispose of these materials safely in Canada. In the United States contact the Housing and Urban Development hotline at 1-800-RID-LEAD or the National Lead Information Center, 1-800-LEAD-FYI.

Paint removal or stripping is probably the most hazardous method of dealing with leaded paints. Disturbing the lead will increase the risk of contamination to the immediate environment and ingestion by the exposed person. It is recommended that such actions be performed only by a qualified individual, particularly if the job is of a large magnitude. Also, heat, sanding, or sandblasting should NEVER be used in lead paint removal. Chemical strippers offer better removal technique for prevention of lead exposure.

When you remove or cover up leaded materials, it is important to realize that the lead is still present where the materials are disposed of or where they are covered up. The covering up or "encapsulation" of leaded paints is not a permanent solution. Continued monitoring and/or testing will remain an important task to prevent any further escape of lead into the immediate environment.

If paint removal is necessary, here are some safety tips to follow. It is particularly important that pregnant women (or women trying to become pregnant) and children are not involved or exposed to the dust or fumes from leaded paint removal. Should the removal be of a large magnitude it is important for children and expectant mothers to stay away from the house until removal and clean-up is completed. Protective clothing, goggles, respirator (not just a face mask) and gloves should be used and cleaned or disposed of immediately after the clean-up. Careful handwashing is a priority. Food and beverages should not be prepared or consumed in the work area. Equally essential as care in removing the leaded paint is adequate clean-up to remove and dispose of the lead particles and dust left in the home after the removal is complete.

In summary, common sense safety principles should be followed in the process of lead removal. More information can be obtained from your ministry of the environment, the U.S. Department of Labor, or your municipal waste management agency.

Soil and dust

Considered by the Centers for Disease Control to be the second most likely source of excessive lead exposure for children, soil contamination is another important consideration when investigating sources of metals in your child's environment. The CDC estimates that as many as 5.9 to 11 million American children are exposed to excessive lead in both soil and dust from multiple sources. Well-travelled roadways are perhaps the biggest culprit for excessive lead contamination. Lead will be present in extremely large amounts in soil contaminated by years, perhaps decades, of leaded car emissions. Certainly any areas that support a nearby highway or freeway will have been contaminated to some degree.

Lead has been used worldwide since the 1930s as an antiknock agent which also improved fuel efficiency of gasoline. The use of leaded gasoline escalated between 1965 and 1975, but then began to fall after 1977. The United States, Canada, Japan, and Australia were among the first nations to begin the switch to unleaded gasoline. By this time, there was enough evidence linking lead from car emissions to extremely detrimental effects on humans, particularly children. Lead continued to be used on a massive scale right up until the mid-1980s, at which time the effects of even low-dose exposure to the metal were beginning to be better understood. Then unleaded gas became mandatory in the United States and Canada. Taiwan, Brazil, South Korea, and many countries in Europe, among others, have also begun phasing out leaded gasoline.

Due to the use of leaded gasoline during the last five to six decades, children playing in their own back yards near busy roads, highways, and freeways may be at serious risk of exposure to very high levels of lead. Test results of soil samples taken from some of the larger freeways in the United States revealed excessive levels of lead contamination up to a one-mile radius surrounding the freeway. The soil sample I took from our house by Mountain Highway, a two-lane highway in North Vancouver, indicated contaminated soil. The bad news is that, despite the fact that these levels exceed British Columbia's Waste Management Act for lead contamination in residential areas, provincial government guidelines do not insist on a clean-up at such levels. On the one hand, these levels are unacceptable . . . on the other hand, no one's going to do anything about it, not even announce the potential health hazard to those living in the contaminated environment. The letter that I received from British Columbia's minister of the environment clearly shows this to be the case:

> It is true that the lead concentration of the single soil sample analyzed exceeds the "Criteria for Managing Contaminated Sites in British Columbia" level A value of 50 ppm [it contained 71 ppm]. However, the level A value is not a residential standard or criteria for soil lead. Level A values represent natural background levels of metals in soils. Furthermore, although an exceedance of level A indicates that the soil is slightly contaminated, remediation of that soil for residential use is not required. The appropriate residential soil quality criteria for lead is level B, 500 ppm. Thus, the ministry would not normally require remediation of any residential soil for lead unless the level B value of 500 ppm was exceeded.

Although the level of blood lead considered to be safe has dropped drastically over the years, our environmental guidelines are not following suit. Although contamination is occurring (and increasing) in industrialized areas every day, governments work with the guidelines that ignore the contamination problem until it exceeds grossly contaminated levels. Even then, some officials are reluctant to act. This is a clear signal that we, as concerned citizens of our industrialized cities, must learn how to protect ourselves from the hazards of excessive lead and metal exposure to our bodies.

Another important potential source of lead in soil and dust is, as mentioned before, the dust and chips of lead-based exterior house paint that fall off older houses and are deposited in adjacent soils. Should these homes be renovated or torn down, more lead will contaminate the soil. It will lie dormant in the soil and continue to accumulate. It may contaminate your children's play area or your garden.

When it gets on the soles of your shoes, it will be walked into the house where it will pose a serious health threat to toddlers who spend their time crawling around on the ground . . . and then put their toys or their hands into their mouths.

If you are suspicious that you may have excessive soil or dust exposure to lead or other metals, you can test soil and dust at most laboratories. Take in about half a cup of soil in a plastic bag. Dust can be taken into a laboratory in a vacuum bag — there are special bags on the market which are frequently used in smelter towns to assess household dust for lead contamination. Your lab can fill you in on the details. If the specimen is found to be contaminated there are several procedures for metal removal or cover-up.

Heavily contaminated soil should be removed, but the area where you dump it will then be contaminated. If certain areas appear to have a less significant amount of lead or other metals, use ground-cover foliage or shrubs to protect children from direct exposure to the metal. Planting grass is also a fairly effective way of controlling lead exposure. Keep in mind that, during dry spells, lead dust will be blown around, contaminating other areas nearby.

Some words of caution: be especially careful to keep children's play areas, sandboxes, and vegetable gardens away from soil contaminated with metals. Any food products grown in metal-rich soil can absorb metals and you will have direct exposure if you consume the contaminated produce.

As previously mentioned, metal-contaminated soil can be tracked into your home on shoes, clothes, toys, etc. It is especially important to practise home hygienic measures for reduction of exposure in metal-rich areas. For example, frequent, thorough vacuuming, dusting with a damp cloth, and damp-mopping floors and hard surfaces are good ideas. Removing shoes before entering the house, and frequent handwashing are also effective in reducing the risk of accidental exposure and ingestion. Handwashing, in fact, is probably the most important step to prevent direct soil/dust metal exposure, particularly for children.

Water and plumbing

Another important thing a family can do to protect their children from excessive metal exposure is to be careful about their consumption of water. Sounds pretty difficult, doesn't it? It's not! If I had known six years ago what I now know about the tap water that I was drinking and preparing my children's bottles and foods with, I might not be in the situation that I am in today with three metal-toxic children. My twins could possibly have been spared their five-year ordeal.

Tap water should be consumed cautiously. The U.S. Environmental Protection Agency (EPA) estimates that drinking water is responsible for approximately 10 to 20 percent of the lead exposure in children. They estimate that about 20 percent of the population is exposed to high levels of lead in their drinking water.

In 1986, amendments to the Safe Drinking Water Act in the United States banned the use of lead pipes and lead solder in plumbing. Canada followed suit. Due to the fact that lead is such a malleable metal, municipal water authorities used it in the construction of water pipelines in the early 1900s. Some of these lead pipes are still present in older water supply systems. Lead pipes were also used in the plumbing of many homes before the 1930s. And despite the ban on lead pipes and the replacement of copper pipes in household plumbing, plumbers were soldering with lead solder up until 1986. (This ban didn't take effect in some parts of the United States until 1988.) Lead in lesser amounts can also be found as a component of some water faucets used in household plumbing. Other metals may be found in plumbing pipes as well.

Along with the lead hazards of plumbing, lead and metal

particles can also leach into a water supply from dumpsites containing lead batteries, or can be added to the water supply in the form of airborne particles emitted from leaded fuel and smelters.

Certain water conditions also affect how much metal is leached out of pipes. While hard (alkaline) water is known to coat pipes and solder with a layer of minerals which makes the pipe or solder less corrosive, thereby reducing the amount of metal leached from these sources, soft (acidic) water does just the opposite. Acidic water has a greater capacity to ionize or mobilize metal out of pipes and solder. The addition of acid rain to water sources will affect the pH. Lime and/or other minerals have long been added to municipal water supplies to control acidity.

Perhaps the simplest, most inexpensive method to reduce accidental exposure to excessive lead and other heavy metals in your tap water is to run the water for about one minute before consuming it. This will clear from the water line any metals that have leached out of the plumbing while the water sat idle in the pipes. An even better method is to run the water until it comes out very cold. When the water runs especially cold it is the water from the water main, not from your house plumbing. This water is unlikely to be contaminated as heavy metals are usually much less concentrated at this point. These simple precautions are inexpensive and are a fairly effective and efficient practice to reduce ingestion of metal from tap water.

Water filtering devices have recently hit the market in a big way. Most can eliminate virtually all the lead and heavy metals that accumulate in tap water. An extremely good example of this type of device is a reverse osmosis water filtering system. Unfortunately, these cost anywhere from CDN$400 up, though they are a worthwhile investment in your health if you can afford it, and they make your water taste and smell great.

Many simpler, less expensive models are available from

health food stores, drugstores, department stores, etc. It is important to check each product's write-up in *Consumer Reports* or similar magazines. Some do not remove all metals, or do not remove them in satisfactory quantities; others boast excellent lead-filtering properties but may contaminate the first few litres or gallons of water with other harmful elements from their filtering system. One such model was described to me by a company which tested filtering devices. The representative told me that, although the lead filtering capabilities were demonstrated to be almost 100 percent effective, the first four litres of water filtered contained elevated levels of silver, another neurotoxin, that was being flushed from the filter unit. Once the first four litres were flushed through, the water was in excellent shape.

A significant piece of information when you're deciding which type of filtering device to buy (or even which method would be better — running tap water until cold *vs.* purchasing a filter) is a tap water analysis. Generally analysis by a certified laboratory for lead costs about CDN$25 to CDN$50. Each additional metal you test for costs extra. There are home test kits available that will perform a rough measure of lead, but these test kits do not always give an accurate account of the concentration present.

Even people in rural communities or those relying upon well water should be concerned about acidic or polluted water, and metals leached out of plumbing. People who drink well water should also be aware that the submersible pumps used in some wells can corrode and introduce massive quantities of lead into their water. I know of a case of severe lead poisoning from such a pump involving a woman in a rural area on Pender Island, British Columbia. A blood test showed acute (recent) exposure to extremely elevated quantities of lead. When the pump in her well was dismantled, it was found that the entire cuff of the lead gasket from the pump had eroded and was disintegrating.

For more details and information on lead and laboratory

testing, the EPA has provided a Safe Drinking Water hotline for the U.S.: 1-800-426-4791. In Canada contact your public health officials.

Now stop to think about the water that you and your family have ingested in the course of a day. You might start your morning off by preparing baby formula with that first blast of metal-rich morning tap water. Even worse, you might sterilize it by boiling, further concentrating lead or other heavy metals, before using it to prepare your baby's formula, juice, or food. Or, like me, you might pull out a package of decaffeinated coffee and make a nice fresh pot of lead-rich coffee. After a good strong cup of morning brew, you then breast-feed your baby. Most of the lead that you just consumed is eventually going to pass into your breast milk and your baby will absorb it into its body tissues. If you are pregnant, lead from that tainted brew passes through the placenta to your unborn baby. If I had known just this piece of information before I had children . . .

Anybody who thinks that their plumbing couldn't possibly be a problem should remember what I said about lead-based paint and older houses. Just because there is now a ban on lead pipes and plumbing doesn't mean that lead pipes no longer exist. Many houses built before the 1950s had lead pipes in their plumbing, and homes built after that had copper pipes with lead solder. Both can contaminate water supplies. More recent plumbing installations can contain significant quantities of other heavy metals.

And bear in mind what my local health officer told me when he said our drinking water poses no health threat. He concluded that our tap water was safe and my kids couldn't have been exposed to excess lead from our tap water — unless, of course, we had consumed it right from the tap. Well, no kidding. What do most people do (especially before 1985 when there were no public warnings about such health dangers)? When even health officials won't drink the water from our taps, we should all be concerned.

Pottery and lead crystal

Another common source of metal exposure for children (and adults) is pottery, ceramic, and crystal dishware. Glazes found on some pottery items and ceramics can contain extremely high levels of lead and other metals, particularly on items from some foreign countries. Lead-glazed pottery from Mexico, China, and developing nations has been found in many cases to have been inadequately fired. The result is lead which leaches into the food or beverage served in the dish. When food or beverages served or stored in such a piece of pottery are eaten, metal poisoning can occur, particularly if the food or beverage is acidic (*i.e.*, tea, coffee, tomato-based). Acidic conditions are prime conditions for lead leaching. Brightly glazed pottery or ceramics are most often found to be a problem. Lead crystal is not exempt from the effects of lead leaching either, especially if it is used to store acidic fluids. If you have any suspicion about a product, refrain from using it for consumption of food or beverages.

Since 1971 American manufacturers have been required to fire their earthenware pottery, ceramics, and china at temperatures that make lead glazes relatively impervious. Many other countries follow this example, and European and Japanese products are generally well-fired, but despite the research and knowledge that such a hazard exists there are still exceptions and many countries still produce items which do not meet the United States Food and Drug Administration Safety Guidelines. The FDA estimates that about 300 million pieces of porcelain sold in the U.S. each year contain levels of lead that would be considered excessive, even by the old standards for lead in porcelain. Buyer beware!

Even pottery which initially tests safe for lead content can begin to release lead after the piece becomes old and worn from continuous washings or is damaged, cracked, or chipped. Such pieces can be responsible for releasing many times the acceptable level of lead. Discard such pieces. As they become worn or damaged, the potential for more leaching of lead increases.

Another good rule is never store food or fluids in pottery, ceramic, lead crystal, or porcelain containers. You can never tell for sure (unless you test the article) just how much lead might be present. Incidentally, I recently spoke with a laboratory director who relayed a story to me. An older woman who had travelled through Europe came back with many little souvenirs. One of them was a beautiful teapot which she used to make her daily tea. After some months she became extremely ill. Her doctors ran all types of tests on her but nothing was conclusive. Despite the test results her health continued to deteriorate and she became bedridden. All she could drink was tea, and her doting husband dutifully continued to bring her her tea in bed. After more unsuccessful testing it suddenly struck her husband that perhaps the pot was leaching lead into the beverage; after all, the more tea she drank, the sicker she became. Sure enough, after the pot was tested at a certified lab, the results revealed extremely high levels of lead being released. The woman stopped drinking tea out of that pot and her health gradually began to improve.

Foods and beverages / canned goods

Considered to be the most common route of lead exposure for adults, food can be contaminated by various means: from the soil in the fields, from emissions of farm equipment, or from motor vehicle emissions when a farm is close to heavily travelled roads. Food can be contaminated at the processing stage by machinery and lead-soldering in pipes or containers, or at the cooking stage when it is washed or cooked in lead-contaminated water, handled by unwashed hands, or prepared on an unclean surface.

Before 1980, more than 90 percent of metal cans were lead-soldered. These cans usually have a raised seam along the side. After 1980 the United States Food and Drug Administration along with the food processors agreed to voluntarily phase out lead solder from cans. This did not apply to imported foods as the phase-out was voluntary. Even today you can still find cans, usually imported, that are lead-soldered. *Consumer Reports* estimated in 1989 that a quarter of imported cans continue to be lead-soldered.

Batteries and recycled oil

Large storage batteries and engine oil are two sources of metal exposure that are commonly overlooked. Especially for adults, battery-breaking operations are sources of excessive lead exposure to the workers who break down the batteries into smaller components and then sort these components. The lead pieces are often melted down in blast furnaces which emit contaminated gases, so workers are exposed to large quantities of lead, along with toxic amounts of acid. Many cases of acute lead poisoning have been recorded in such factories. Headaches and palsied limbs are frequent symptoms of this source of exposure to adults. There have also been reports of metal poisoning within residential communities that are located close to these plants.

The CDC reports that many children are exposed to lead from batteries and, more frequently, recycled oil. Recycled oil is usually not re-refined for motor oil, but is sold to be burned as fuel in industrial boilers and furnaces used to heat office buildings and apartments. This causes an increase in emission of airborne lead particles into the atmosphere.

In summary

Due to the serious health threat that metals impose on our young children it is wise to modify your home and imme-

diate environment so that it is safe for your children. Be sure
to check old paint for damage, flaking, or chipping. Regularly monitor these potential problem areas. Testing your
paint may also help put your mind at ease if you suspect it
might be a source of lead. Follow lead-safe protocols when
renovating.

Everyone should be concerned enough about their water
supply to establish safe practices for water consumption in
their household. You might want to test your water for your
own peace of mind. Regardless of whether you test it or not,
make sure you run the tap water for at least fifteen seconds
before drinking the water. Otherwise, purchase a water filtering device which is effective for lead and heavy metal removal. Never use hot tap water for baby formulas, cooking
vegetables, beverages, or other uses when preparing food for
ingestion. Hot water is more likely to leach lead out of solder
and pipes.

Feeding your children a diet which is low in fat and high
in calcium and iron will help them avoid excessive lead absorption into their body tissues. Calcium competes with lead
in the bowel and prevents excessive absorption of lead into
the bloodstream. Avoid metal cookware, particularly aluminum. Avoid using aluminum wrappers or containers with
acidic fluids and foodstuffs. Avoid tinned foodstuffs, particularly those containing acidic substances. Whenever possible, use fresh produce and wash it thoroughly. Consider
adding daily vitamin and mineral supplements to your diet,
particularly if you are not sure your children's nutritional
intake is adequate.

Test suspicious soil or use a ground cover to keep the areas
in question from being a direct source of exposure to children. Remove heavily contaminated areas. Maintain some
good home hygiene practices such as frequent, effective
handwashing, particularly before food consumption.

Avoid ceramic food containers for storing foods and liq-
uids, especially foods that are highly acidic, and use crystal

dishes only for serving food, not for food storage. Whenever possible, check labels on pottery for lead content before purchasing an item. If in doubt, don't use the piece for food.

If you are in a high-risk occupation or live near an industrial area that is highly contaminated, be aware and take as many precautions as you can. If you are unsure, test yourself, your family, perhaps your drinking water, and even the soil around you. Wear protective clothing and masks where required. Avoid handling toxic metals by hand as your skin is the body's largest absorptive organ. If you work in an industry where heavy metal contamination is a problem, be careful with your work clothes. Bag them before bringing them into your car or into your home for cleaning. If you are in a high-risk situation, have your hair and urine tested at least annually.

If you are a woman of childbearing age, arrange to be tested before you have babies.

If you have an illness similar to any of those described in this book for which nobody has been able to give you a reasonable explanation, and where, despite various interventions, no benefits are being obtained, suspect toxicity as a reasonable alternative. Be particularly careful with children at least up until the age of six, during which time there is the greatest amount of brain growth and development.

By educating yourself and your family, and following some simple common-sense rules, you can avoid accidental, insidious ingestion of lead and many other heavy metals which do not belong in the human body. Public awareness is extremely important for everybody. This is not an isolated problem for a few areas. It is an international problem. Every country is affected to some degree. The health risks and sources of potential metal exposure can no longer be ignored.

11

Getting the Lead Out

Shortly after Cam and Brett were diagnosed with metal poisoning, as we started to work on this book, Zigurts told me the story of Ignaz Semmelweis, a Hungarian physician who worked in a Viennese hospital in the mid 1800s. The perceptive Dr. Semmelweis noticed that there was a higher incidence of postpartum infection in women who were being examined by physicians and residents as opposed to those who were examined by nurses and designated ward staff. Dr. Semmelweis observed that physicians who had the highest patient mortality rates were examining women right after performing post-mortem examinations in the pathology labs. He concluded that these physicians were transporting bacteria from their dissections and contaminating relatively healthy but vulnerable patients. Although there was a lot of resistance, he persuaded these physicians to wash their hands prior to treating the women. As a result, the mortality rates dropped to less than 1 percent from 10 to 20 percent.

After presenting his findings to the Vienna Medical Society, he encountered such opposition that the medical director of his hospital demoted him. He left Vienna, returned to Budapest, and eventually, as a result of the ridicule, Semmelweis suffered a nervous breakdown and was sent to an asylum where he died, ironically, of a blood-borne infection.

Zigurts told me this story as an example of how difficult it is for the medical establishment to change — how difficult it is to introduce new ideas. We were already meeting resistance to our ideas about metal poisoning and detoxification from doctors, government medical officers, and politicians. I have to admit I was flabbergasted by the reluctance of doctors in particular to take our information seriously. It was obvious the parents of the affected children had no difficulty recognizing this problem once the information was made available to them.

It's not as if the toxicity of heavy metals, particularly lead, is unproven. Nor is the knowledge that they cause neurological compromise a new discovery. Our observation that the symptoms of metal toxicity can be mistaken for the symptoms of autism *is* new. Or maybe we have discovered that some cases of autism will respond to heavy metal detoxification. But I wasn't prepared for doctors to dismiss the idea without at least exploring the possibility that metals were affecting children in their care.

Zigurts was able to give me some explanation for resistance in the medical field. He pointed out that because new ideas are understood and studied by relatively few people, the uninformed majority, through lack of knowledge and awareness, will generally oppose new knowledge. The information must be documented, recorded, and perhaps practised by a few insightful medical practitioners or researchers before a significant number start to acquire and use the knowledge, and resistance is overcome.

Then there is the paradox of a medical education in which information is handed down from "authorities" while, at the same time, student doctors are encouraged to maintain an open, inquisitive mind and aspire to discover new things. Can a system that is built on indoctrinating physicians with established beliefs be flexible enough to accept new ideas emanating from the rank and file?

Finally, physicians are much more willing to accept the information derived from a double-blind university-based drug study that is sponsored by a multi-national drug company than observations made by practising clinicians.

Fortunately a number of leading physicians and researchers are aware of the profession's lopsided nature, and welcome new ideas, allow their dissemination in medical and scientific journals, and encourage further research. Unfortunately, however, anyone who does record any new observations or proposes new ideas can still anticipate a period of "expert" resistance.

Some of the parents Zigurts and I talked to about lead poisoning and detoxification came back to us and said that their family doctors or pediatricians told them chelation was harmful to children. These doctors were sometimes visibly angry that this testing was being carried out on their patients, but I am not aware that any of these physicians suspected or tested for heavy metals in the children despite symptoms suggestive of metal toxicity (*i.e.*, colic, diarrhea, poor appetite, anxiety, pica, and language delay). I can't tell you with certainty why many of these doctors were so alarmed at this avenue of investigation. None offered any adequate explanation, just resistance and disbelief. However, I do know that chelation therapy is currently regarded as controversial in the medical profession when it is used for the treatment of atherosclerosis — hardening of the arteries. Some of these physicians did not appear to realize that chelation therapy is not a controversial issue in the treatment of lead toxicity and lead encephalopathy. It is the only treatment for removal of excess heavy metals from the human body and has been acknowledged as such in the *New England Journal of Medicine*, the Bible of medical journals. The College of Physicians and Surgeons of British Columbia also affirms the use of chelation for the removal of excess heavy metals in the human body. In a 1992 public statement the college reiterated its position that "the appropriate use of chelation to treat lead poisoning is approved by the Council." When I contacted the registrar for the college's position on chelation, and indicated that some doctors were reluctant to use it to test for heavy metal toxicity, he appeared concerned that college members were missing this diagnosis and wrote, "Since recognition of the possibility of lead poisoning should lie within the realm of capabilities of the vast majority of licensed medical practitioners, it would be appropriate for the College to pursue your concerns with those whom you are speaking of. It would be desirable for the College to obtain the necessary information to evaluate whether they dealt with your children's problems appropriately. If failure to diagnose existing lead and other heavy metal toxicities is occurring, it should be taken up with the doctors involved. For us to do that, we will need you to identify those doctors."

This brings me back to a point that I made earlier. Testing for lead and other heavy metals should be part of the initial diagnosis of a child who presents with the problems described in this book. However, I don't believe hindsight is a good tool to use to confront the medical profession or establish blame or negligence. It *is* a good tool to use to enable us to avoid repeating past mistakes. I didn't feel that it was ethical or beneficial to anyone to turn physicians in. I always felt that my children's doctors were looking out for their best interests. Besides, it is the college's job to ensure the medical profession is up-to-date and educated in current medicine — not mine.

As a mother of three children whose lives may have been wasted, I am thankful I found a general practitioner who had developed the knowledge and skills to diagnose and treat this problem. He acknowledges that two years earlier he would have missed the diagnosis for lack of knowledge.

It is not just the medical profession that is slow to adopt new ideas. My experience with the local health officer and politicians revealed a frightening lack of interest and concern from those in a position to institute education and awareness of these issues. There are no doubt multitudes of bureaucratic implications when dealing with a health hazard like heavy metals. I suspect that the failure of health officials to deal with (or want to get involved in) this issue could stem from a reluctance to address the social, economic, health, and environmental implications. For example, what is the government's responsibility for those children suffering various degrees of mental impairment or retardation caused by metal poisoning? Who would be responsible for compensation and clean-up — government, or the industry that caused the pollution? Who would pay for treatment and education or care of the affected children? In my encounters with the medical officers and provincial politicians I didn't even get as far as these questions, as they all denied there was a problem.

Both my children's pediatrician and my family physician suggested I contact the municipal medical health officer to alert him to the presence of lead and other toxic metals in our area. I sent him: certified laboratory test results indicating a water sample from my former home which contained 9.6 times the acceptable level of lead; a soil sample from my former home which indicated lead contamination that was 42 percent higher than the acceptable level for a residential zone; my children's laboratory results that indicated they were excreting huge quantities of heavy metals; and anecdotal evidence of the incredible changes that I, and everybody else working with my children, had witnessed. The health officer maintained that this was probably just an isolated incident and didn't warrant investigating. When I told him that many other children in the area had also suffered from neurological problems and subsequent testing for body burden of heavy metals indicated that they, too, were excreting excess quantities of lead and other metals, he stated that he would like to see their results. However, he said he would only base an investigation on blood lead levels. He was only interested in elevated blood lead levels, even though blood is not a good measure of chronic toxicity. As my children were victims of chronic heavy metal toxicity, I would never be able to provide a blood lead result high

enough to warrant an investigation according to his criteria
. . . despite all of the other pieces of evidence.

After several frustrating months dealing with the health
officer, I went a few steps higher and wrote a letter outlining
my concerns to the provincial health minister. This letter —
which I copied to the federal ministry of health and provincial ministries of the environment and social services, to the
premier of British Columbia, to the North Shore and Vancouver health officers, and to the B.C. College of Physicians
and Surgeons — was signed by eleven parents of metal-toxic
children and eight childcare providers who had worked with
the affected children. We carefully laid out the case for
screening young children for metals.

> As it appears that children are most vulnerable to the
> ingestion of lead and other heavy metals during the first
> five to six years of development, it is reasonable to as-
> sume that many more children today are being ad-
> versely and perhaps permanently affected by this
> problem. Our children's health care interests have been
> sadly neglected and, as a result, some of them are now
> the victims of varying degrees of permanent neurologi-
> cal damage (*i.e.*, mental retardation). Our crucial ques-
> tion at this time is "who will assume the responsibility
> of ensuring that other children with similar sympto-
> mology will be given the opportunity for lead and other
> heavy metal screening?" In addition and more impor-
> tantly, "who will take the responsibility to ensure that
> what is described to be a completely preventable phe-
> nomenon will not continue to happen to our young
> developing Canadian children?" These damaged chil-
> dren are a huge drain of social resources and funding.
> Ongoing extensive social supports and services are re-
> quired for these children when neurological damage of
> chronic lead and other heavy metal toxicities has oc-
> curred and when the opportunity for PROPER testing

and treatment of chronic metal poisoning is neither readily available nor accessible. We feel that this is of utmost importance and needs to be addressed immediately, regardless of the political, financial, and/or other ramifications that this might entail.

We cited the Centers for Disease Control statistic that one in six preschool children could be affected, mentioned the United States lead prevention program, and the Royal Society of Canada's Commission on Lead in the Environment, and attached supporting documents and lab results.

In response, Paul Ramsey, British Columbia's health minister, wrote:

> While it is clear that people are now more concerned about the effects of lead than ever before, significant reductions in children's blood lead levels have been achieved through the phase-out of lead in gasoline and through changes in food processing . . . I am concerned by your statement that your children were poisoned by lead and other heavy metals at your former residence. As you have not enclosed the results of any blood lead testing in your children, neither I, nor Ministry of Health staff can offer any comment on this matter. Blood lead is the accepted measure for determining whether or not children have had excessive exposure to lead. If an elevated blood level is found, further testing may be warranted to assess the amount of lead deposited in bones.

Just great! The health minister sent me a letter citing today's drop in blood levels of lead due to government interventions, despite the fact that I emphasized in my letter to him, and provided documented data verifying the conclusion that blood levels are inaccurate for measuring the body burden of lead and other metals in cases of chronic exposure.

I decided that the health minister needed further educating. After all, he had been the parliamentary secretary to the ministry of forests until a few months earlier and was only recently appointed to the health ministry. What did he really know about health? It was obvious that he was responding with information supplied to him from his own resources — possibly the health officers from the North Shore and Vancouver. And look at where we got with that. In my next correspondence I re-emphasized the inaccuracy of blood lead levels.

> In my letter it was made extremely clear that I was not talking about blood levels of lead. Information that I sent to you that has been documented by highly regarded and acclaimed medical bodies (*i.e.*, the Royal Society of Canada, McGill University, Harvard University, Albert Einstein College, etc.) indicates that BLOOD LEAD LEVELS DO NOT REFLECT BODY BURDEN OF LEAD. THEY ARE GOOD INDICATORS OF RECENT EXPOSURE ONLY, AS OPPOSED TO POOR INDICATORS OF LONG-TERM, CHRONIC EXPOSURE. Children with neurological damage are subject to CHRONIC toxicity — not acute toxicity! You, of all people, need to be aware of this! It is for this reason that blood lead level results that you indicated to be important in your return letter have no relation to my letter of October 30/93.

I added, "Your comment that 'incidents of lead poisoning are rare' is somewhat accurate. This is mostly due to the fact that few are looking for it adequately here! I would like to suggest to you that (1) the definition of lead poisoning is somewhat of a 'grey' area which makes it very difficult to assess, and, therefore, very easy for the medical profession to ignore, and, (2) there are many cases of lead poisoning, it's just that few physicians are actually looking for it and adequately testing and diagnosing these incidents!"

Soon after receiving the response from Ramsey, I received a letter from the federal health minister, Diane Marleau. Her letter acknowledged that the responsibility for reducing the health risks of lead was shared between all levels of government but, most interesting of all, she commented that despite these efforts, "problem situations" such as mine do occur. She also stated, "This is a clear signal that we must not abandon our efforts in dealing with lead toxicity."

So the federal government was the first and only level of Canadian government to agree that metal poisoning does, in fact, continue to be a problem, that these situations do occur, and that we must continue to work on solving this problem.

But what is being done? We fear that our experiences with the medical profession and politicians are not that unusual, and parents, educators, childcare workers, environmentalists, and others are going to have to speak out strongly to make some changes in the way we treat children and their environment.

Change has happened before. For years the automotive industry built cars that burned massive amounts of leaded gasoline despite the fact that there was technology around that could build more fuel-efficient, less polluting engines. It was not until the economics of pollution were appreciated in California that the state government legislated the toughest standards for fuel emissions in the United States and countries began banning the use of lead in gasoline.

Yes, lead has been removed from gasoline in recent years. It was reduced in, and then banned from, paints. Plumbing codes have changed and so have standards in food canning and production. Pottery and ceramic glazing is monitored. But even so, lead from decades of car emissions is still present in the soil. Leaded paint in older housing did not simply disappear. It will continue to be a problem until it is removed or covered. Lead has not disappeared from water just because lead solder was banned in the plumbing industry.

Our water district still issues warnings to run water for at least fifteen seconds before use, suggesting it is otherwise unfit for human consumption.

Industry continues to use an ever-increasing supply of lead and other heavy metals due to their malleability, their resistance to many kinds of corrosion, their near indestructibility, and their abundance and easy availability. We must also be aware that we are part of a global village, connected by the atmosphere and by the ocean. We in North America have been releasing lead and other toxic metals into this environment for at least the past century and now newly industrialized countries are adding their share of pollution. The half-life of lead and other heavy metals is such that they will continue to be in soil, housing, air, and water, and will pose a potential health problem, for decades to come.

Can we clean it up? Unfortunately, and not surprisingly, there appears to be a huge price tag attached to any clean-up of lead and other heavy metals in our environment. It costs a lot of money to test for, remedy, and prevent further metal exposure in a community, let alone an entire continent. And we must not be so naive as to assume that government and industry will leap forward to help us. The companies that mine and use lead and other heavy metals often will not admit that their products pose a health hazard. Understandably, they do not want to pay money for clean-up and safety standards, or lose money by producing fewer items or using more expensive materials. And the replacement materials can be just as hazardous as the metals they replace, as, for example, when cadmium replaces lead in piping.

But look at it this way: we as parents, children, individuals, are paying the price through ill health, lost potential, and medical and care costs. Why shouldn't the mining and manufacturing industries carry their cost of the burden by helping to prevent childhood poisoning? If you are in a contaminated community, join with other parents of affected children to pressure local industry and government to remove or cover up polluted soil. Let the federal government know that you don't think industry should get away with pollution.

Considering the cost — in time and money — of a clean-up, it is probably wise not to count on its happening quickly. We should work for increased public awareness of the sources and dangers of exposure to heavy metals for young children at the same time as we are working to remove these sources. Information is available about acute exposure; more parents must be informed of the dangers of chronic exposure.

Fortunately I'm finding that this information gets around in spite of official resistance. Parents in North Vancouver and as far away as Nova Scotia were able to get in touch with me; colleagues from Canada, the United States, and New Zealand approach Zigurts because they've heard of his work with lead-toxic children. In the midst of my correspondence with B.C.'s health minister I was contacted by a social worker from the provincial ministry of social services who called me in for a meeting to discuss my children. She was impressed by the changes she was hearing about, and mentioned that she was aware that many other families she was dealing with had witnessed exciting and encouraging changes in the condition of their mentally handicapped children after commencing the detoxification program. She said the ministry was distributing the information I had given them and was encouraging other clients to investigate this avenue in cases that were suggestive of metal toxicity. They were also surprised at the amount of current information available regarding metal toxicity and wondered why it had been missed for so long. Too bad this woman wasn't the minister of health.

After we've educated parents, politicians, and doctors about chronic toxicity, we can start to identify and treat children who have been poisoned. I'm not just talking about children who are grossly affected, as my twins were. There is a huge grey area in the definition of what constitutes metal toxicity. Current research shows that problems are definitely occurring at levels of exposure previously considered safe. In October 1991 the Centers for Disease Control launched a campaign to increase public awareness of the seriousness of lead poisoning, and to encourage efforts to recognize and prevent this hazard. They remarked:

Since virtually all children are at risk for lead poisoning, a phase of universal screening is recommended . . . Efforts need to be increasingly focused on preventing lead poisoning before it occurs. This will require communitywide environmental interventions, as well as educational and nutritional campaigns . . . Screening and medical treatment of poisoned children will remain critically important until the environmental sources most likely to poison children are eliminated . . . This will require a shared responsibility among many public and private agencies . . . Healthcare providers will need to phase in virtually universal screening of children . . . In February 1991, the Department of Health and Human Services released a "Strategic Plan for the Elimination of Childhood Lead Poisoning" (HHS, 1991). This plan describes the first five years of a twenty-year society-wide effort to eliminate this disease. It places highest priority on addressing the children at greatest risk for lead poisoning. The Department of Housing and Urban Development (HUD, 1990) and the Environmental Protection Agency (EPA, 1991) have both released plans dealing with the elimination of lead hazards. To eliminate this disease will require tremendous effort from all levels of government as well as the private sector, but we believe that the benefits to society will be well worth it. We look forward to the day when childhood lead poisoning is no longer a public health problem.

Even children who appear healthy can have high levels of

lead in their blood, so the CDC recommends that all children be tested for lead poisoning at one year old. Testing should be done at six months old if your home is known to have lead in it, or if you live in an older building. It further recommends that all children older than one year have their blood tested every couple of years — every year if your home contains lead. (Unfortunately, they don't recommend doing anything much about it unless the lead level is 10 µg/dl or higher.)

Many pediatric doctors have recently been quoted as saying that we must not ignore the CDC statements — lead is the number one health hazard to young children.

Herbert Needleman and Philip J. Landrigan are two doctors who have studied the effects of lead and other environmental hazards on children. In their book *Raising Children Toxic Free* they estimate that the cost of caring for a child with lead poisoning is, conservatively, US$4600, and there may be 3 or 4 million children who need this care, shooting costs into the billions of dollars.

Those are the American figures. In my province alone the ministry of social services announced in December 1993 that about 2800 children across the province were in special needs daycare programs at a cost of CDN$24 million annually. (This represents an annual cost of approximately CDN$8600 per child for preschool alone.) December 1994 figures revealed over 3000 children were now enrolled in this program. Children in the special needs program have mental, physical, communicative, or behavioral disabilities. This is the type of program that Cam and Brett and many of the other children described in this book were involved in.

This is only the cost of children's daycare programs. Many of these children will require expensive medications like Ritalin, which costs in the area of CDN$600 a year or more, perhaps for life, and will need special educational assistants throughout their school career at a cost in excess of CDN$15,000 per year for a full-time aide. They may also require behavioral consultants, childcare workers, and speech and language pathologists, not to mention the never-ending visits to medical specialists and their batteries of expensive tests. They will likely receive a handicapped pension as an adult from age eighteen till death. They may incur extra governmental expenses for housing programs, medical programs, job training programs, and childcare, youthcare, and adultcare workers for ongoing support and assistance throughout their entire lifetimes. One estimate that we heard of the current costs of supporting an autistic child (which, keep in mind, might actually be a metal-toxic child) were in excess of CDN$1 million over the course of his or her lifetime. Do you know how much it costs to test and treat a child for metal toxicity? Only about CDN$200 to CDN$400. Imagine how much money we would save if we were able to improve an autistic child's condition enough that he might need only half of the usual services.

During the course of my battle with municipal and provincial politicians and reluctant doctors, many friends and relatives asked me, "Why can't you just be happy that you found out what was causing your children's problems and forget about it?" There are many reasons why I choose not to forget about it. The one that occurs to me almost every day of my life is the fact that there was a time when my children were so demented from metal toxicity that I was making plans to terminate my family.

I know that my children were all born "normal." They were delightful as newborns. We invested our whole lives into these children and banked our future on them. We had dreams and plans for them. They had the gift of life, love, and financial security . . . they could have done anything. But they were the victims of lead and other metals which caused mental deterioration and brain damage. Knowing that this same scenario is occurring in many other households is disturbing. Knowing that it could be prevented is mind-boggling. By writing this book, and battling officials, we want to bring this silent menace out into the open, to let as many parents as possible know it's a danger to their chil dren, and, we hope, to put industry, the medical profession, and government on notice that we're angry and we're not going to put up with this anymore.

Again, we must emphasize, let's never be so naive as to assume that authorities will leap forward to help us. It is obvious that little or no interest in pursuing this area of health in our young children will come from industry or government without public exposure and demand. Government works to end acute lead exposure by monitoring blood levels, reducing lead contamination from paint, gasoline, etc., and improving public awareness of this health hazard. However, there is a huge area that is being completely missed, or perhaps ignored — chronic toxicity. Due to the fact that government and health officials refuse to look at anything other than blood levels of lead, there will never be an investigation into the chronic toxicity of children who are victims of continuous exposure to lead and other heavy metals during their infancy. We know that there are many victims of such exposure. We have to find them. Maybe we should decide at what stage we want to start paying for this problem — now, while we can salvage some of these children, or later on, when they require constant social and financial support. It will cost big bucks to clean up. It will cost big bucks to develop and implement screening and treatment programs. So how are we going to do it? Can we afford to do it?

My question is, can we afford not to do it? Little people eventually become big people. Metal-toxic children do not develop mentally, socially, physically into functioning adults. Instead of contributing to society they need society to support them. And heavy metals also contribute to the occurrence of chronic diseases like hypertension, heart disease, etc. in adults. What is and what will be the social and economic cost of a poisoned generation?

Epilogue

This is not the end of our account . . . it is merely the beginning. A beginning for Cameron and Brett, twin boys who had been diagnosed at age three as children with attention deficit hyperactivity disorder and autistic tendencies. They have now completed eighteen months of deleading their body tissues with six rounds of chelation therapy plus mineral supplementation, and are progressing extremely well. They are certainly no longer attention deficit nor hyperactive. Out of fourteen classical signs of autism that they once possessed, they have dropped twelve of the characteristics completely. The remaining two are not as noticeable whereas prior to treatment, they were grossly exaggerated.

At age three, Cameron and Brett were prescribed Ritalin, then Anafranil, and eventually the Anafranil was compounded with Clonidine. Since their first chelation procedure they have not needed any medications at all for their previously diagnosed disorders. Their quality of life has improved dramatically. The twins now love to sit at the table with the family for meals. Their appetites have vastly improved. They have excellent eye contact and much better concentration abilities. They are happy and playful almost all of the time. Fecal smearing is a thing of the past. It has not occurred once since their first deleading treatment. We can finally have company again!

Cam and Brett are now six years old and in Grade 1 at our local public school. The boys are assisted by two teacher's aides who help them follow the majority of the regular Grade 1 curriculum with a large focus on language, social, and fine motor skills. Both children are making rapid, steady progress, and are continuously developing more of these important skills. Although they seem to have some trouble with auditory discrimination (distinguishing sounds), their words are becoming much clearer every day and their comprehension of spoken words is also improving. Brett can read words and books on his own, and is constantly improving his language comprehension while becoming familiar with written words. Both boys appear to have hyperlexia — the ability to identify and learn word meaning (and therefore improve comprehension) through the use of written words. Cam, although appearing to follow four to five months behind Brett in most academic skills, has definite pre-reading skills and is currently able to read most words in his Grade 1 reader. Their fine motor skills have improved tremendously. They can eat with cutlery now, they can print with a pencil, cut with scissors, catch a ball.

The twins are both eagerly and happily participating in school. Although they do not demonstrate the same level of social or academic skills as their same-aged peers, they are making impressive gains on a daily basis. They have a much longer attention span and can stay on task for long periods of time. Due to the loss of the first five years of social and cognitive gains in their lives, it would be unrealistic to presume that they could ever catch up to their peers. And knowing that heavy metals do cause some permanent damage to delicate brain tissues, we are aware that some of the damage is irreversible. However, their potential now shines through — we have something definite and positive to work with.

Despite the fact that their behavior is continuously improving, the twins continue to be "drawn into" or overstimulated by fast-moving or spinning objects. However, they react with much less pronounced self-stimulating behaviors such as hand flicking and/or facial grimacing. Also, when these behaviors do occur I can point it out to them, tell them to relax, and they'll generally stop the unusual behavior and start laughing about it. Gone are the days of running out to grab at the spinning tires of cars or reaching out to touch the train as it speeds by. They finally have a sense of danger.

The twins can sit and watch a full movie and understand most of it. They can watch shows on television with the rest of the family — not just the TV test pattern. They read books from start to finish and take special care of their books. No more shredding. Once again we are able to have glass dishes. Eggs are safe in our refrigerator. We have furniture that isn't damaged. They can go into a person's house to visit without destroying it. They wear clothes now! We have children over to play and, yes, the twins play appropriately with toys. They even request the toys that they want to buy and tell us what stores to find them in. They are finally invited to birthday parties for children from school, and Cam and Brett are planning their own birthday party.

These rapid changes are amazing to the medical community and anybody involved with special needs childhood development and education. These things just don't happen for children with diagnoses like Cam and Brett had.

Although there are still many unknowns, many questions that cannot yet be answered regarding Cam and Brett's expected progression, development, and academic abilities, for the first time since they were toddlers I am excited and optimistic about what the future might hold for my twins. They have demonstrated that they have tremendous potential. We now have children that are much more reasonable and attentive. We were once told by a children's specialist that these twins might never talk. They really are talking now. They have meaningful language. Although their comprehension of complex verbal language at this point is poor, they are making impressive gains and their comprehension is improving every day. And there's no reason why it shouldn't continue to do so. The twins are finally able to reason and they are definitely much more capable of learning. Their unusual anxieties and agitation have disappeared. Their eye contact is great. All of this has resulted from removing toxic metals from their body tissues. Their future is certainly looking much brighter, as is the rest of our family's.

I have an incredible respect for and owe a debt of gratitude to Zigurts Strauts, the man responsible for providing the key to my children's extraordinary recovery. He was the only doctor who suspected heavy metal toxicity in my children, and the only doctor who had the knowledge and the willingness to provide suitable testing and treatment for these children and for many other children and adults. He is a remarkable man. He has provided immeasurable help, hope, and relief to so many families in the last few years, he has guided other physicians and shared his experience with those who have asked. Because of this caring, courageous, and open-minded physician and others like him, I know there will be many more successful recoveries to come.

Many neurologically impaired children have now taken the opportunity for adequate lead and other heavy metal screening, and many of the test results are proving to be positive. The final, indisputable proof of metal toxicity is in the child's recovery. Many of these special needs kids are making that incredible recovery. Every day presents a whole new promise for growth and development. Despite the fact that these kids have already lost many important years, their capabilities for accelerated and continued progress now exist as a result of their more stable and logical mental functioning. And, best of all, they are happy children who feel much better about themselves and their newly acquired abilities. There is an astounding new quality to their lives.

With the information available to you in this book, you will have to decide whether your child, or a child that you know, may have encountered excessive heavy metals as an infant that may now be causing neurological damage. Before a child is diagnosed with attention deficit disorder, hyper-activity, learning disabilities, autistic tendencies, or any other disorder that includes some of the symptoms and behaviors that we know can result from metal toxicity, make sure that this testing is done. Pressure your doctor into looking at this information. Give him support and encouragement. Give him this book if you have to. Sometimes taking a "hard copy" of information to a professional is the best way to get his or her attention. Many doctors don't know about the current research in this area. They are still using testing methods known to be ineffective for measuring the body burden of metals. Many aren't even looking at the possibility of other metal toxicities and, given the medical profession's chelation phobia, it is likely that this treatment will not be all that easily accessed. (Patients and medical practitioners interested in specific guidelines and protocols for the treatment of metal toxicity in children should refer to the last page of this book).

After we investigate and treat our own children, it is imperative that we make ourselves more aware of the health risks that these metals pose to all children and adults, and begin to establish some techniques for prevention of accidental heavy metal exposure . . . and I mean on an international level. No country is exempt from the possibility of excessive heavy metal exposure, therefore no children should be exempt from the opportunity of cure. If they are not detected they will become and remain toxic adults. Parents, childcare workers, healthcare workers, industry, and environmentalists must all be involved to make the larger community aware of the danger and the damage done by heavy metals. They will also be essential in the move to prevention to reduce the risks and damage from this type of insidious, degenerative toxicity.

There is no controversy over the fact that lead and other heavy metals are toxic. There are, however, many opposing opinions regarding the safe or acceptable amounts of metal exposure, the type of screening and testing for lead that should be done, and the age at which it should occur. Remember that lead levels previously considered acceptable are no longer thought safe. Extensive testing has shown even small amounts of lead can be extremely harmful, particularly at certain early stages of human development. Prevention is critical, but drastic measures and public awareness are the keys to rectifying the damage that has already been done.

It was once thought that the damage from lead poisoning was irreversible, therefore there was little effort to treat children who were suspected to be toxic. I sure hope we've cleared up that misconception in this book.

Unfortunately, screening, testing, and clean-up do appear to have that never-ending cost component attached. Some people will argue that it must be "financially feasible" to test for lead and other metals but, in the long term, how financially feasible is it to support metal-toxic individuals for the duration of their lives? How socially feasible is it? When looking at the cost factor involving these children's long-term care and support, doesn't it make sense to foot the bill now and avoid having these children needing the extra supports and hidden costs of housing and maintaining mentally handicapped adults when some of it can be prevented? What about the quality of that human life? Don't we owe children the chance of a recovery from what might be an environmental problem which was caused by years of ignorance and neglect? Don't we all deserve a chance at living life to our fullest potential?

It is important, though, to realize that there are other legitimate reasons for behavior problems and mental handicaps. Don't conclude that you have found the answer to your child's problem from reading this book. Metal toxicity will not be the answer for every child experiencing difficulties. However, we know that it will be the answer for many of these children. When we began testing my children for lead,

I was told by trusted professionals that we were pursuing a shot in the dark, that we were looking for answers that weren't there. They will be the first ones to get a copy of this book! It's easier to open one's mind to search for other possibilities, particularly such a well-documented and researched health hazard as lead, than to tar all of these children with the same brush, applying the mentally handicapped label, and then telling the parents to deal with that for the rest of their lives.

In reflecting on my life with my special needs children, I feel great sadness, frustration, and anger. I wish that I had the same knowledge before they were conceived that I have today. It would have saved years of heartache and grief. It would have given me my children, the way they were intended to be, with their full potential as "normal" children and adults. It would have given them the chance to grow and develop as most other children do. I wish that I didn't have to write this story, that somebody else had done it years ago. It might have changed our lives.

On the other hand, I am thrilled to have been an integral part of this investigation. And I'm determined to pass the message on to as many people as possible. We have no choice but to start assessing and dealing with the environmental hazards that have been created and supported by us all. Lead and other heavy metals will not just go away. Neither will their harmful effects on the human body. They will continue to accumulate and cause many more unnecessary problems until we deal with them as a unified group of concerned people. It is clear that we all must educate ourselves and our communities about the harmful affects of lead and other heavy metals in our environment. We must learn to be aware of their presence in our daily activities, to remove them safely and properly dispose of them. Most importantly, we must learn how to protect ourselves and our offspring from the silent ingestion of these toxins.

Something strange happened to me in the summer of 1993, just four months after finding out that my children were metal poisoned. I was walking through a local shopping mall with my sister when we came upon a psychic fair. There were twelve tables set up with a psychic at each table, eleven women and one man. I noticed that the man was looking at me, and I felt compelled to head towards him. I usually don't go for this kind of stuff but I felt energy — something weird was happening and I wanted to see what it was.

When I approached David Cloud's table he told me, "You are involved in something that is going to be far bigger than what you have ever imagined." Then he asked, "Do you know what an alchemist is?"

I responded, "No, not really."

"Well, you were an alchemist in a past life and you're an alchemist now. This has everything to do with what you're onto right now. Pardon the metaphor, but does it mean anything to you when I say you have found a way to transform lead into gold?"

I started to laugh. I told David that I was writing a book about my experience in treating my lead-toxic children and other children from the community suffering from toxic metals. He then advised me, "You're laughing — you find this funny, but you have no idea how big this is . . . it is far bigger than you could ever imagine . . . you have to have the face of humble awe in this pursuit."

David Cloud — I now know that you were absolutely right. This is big! This is a worldwide health epidemic involving innocent young children. And in correcting this epidemic, we are indeed turning lead into gold!

Appendix

What is Autism and Attention Deficit Disorder?

I'd like to take a few pages here to talk about autism. You will have noticed that I refer to children labeled with "autistic tendencies." These children are not truly autistic but display behavior patterns that are common to autism. Infants who are considered too young to accurately diagnose as autistic are fitted with the autistic tendencies label because until they are more fully developed it is difficult to predict how severe these characteristics will be.

Autism is a rare, life-long developmental disability that is believed to be present at birth, and is recognized by age three. The cause is unknown. Some researchers suggest it is a physical problem which affects those parts of the brain that process language and which affect the way in which the brain analyzes information coming from the five senses. Others think it's the result of chemical imbalances in the brain. Some suggest that genetic factors predispose a person to autism, or that certain viruses may be involved. And many think it's the combination of several factors.

Autism occurs in five to twenty children out of every 10,000 births. It is present throughout the world among all races and social classes. Four out of five people with autism are male. In 1994, there were approximately 1000 school-age children with autism in British Columbia.

Some of the behavior characteristics common to autism are ritualistic and rigid patterns of behavior and/or activity. Autistic individuals typically engage in self-stimulatory behaviors such as rocking, hand flicking, spinning, twisting, and other repetitive movement. They are generally difficult to manage and can exhibit frequent temper tantrums and destructive or self-injurious types of behavior like self-biting, headbanging, hair pulling, eye gouging, etc. They often exhibit extremely inconsistent patterns of sensory responses and many appear to have hypo- or hypersensitivities to sight, taste, smell, touch, and/or hearing. They may become distressed by particular sounds or noises or, alternatively, may fail to respond to, or are unable to respond to, words or sounds, often appearing to be deaf. They may be unresponsive to extreme temperatures and may under- or over-react to heat or cold. They frequently exhibit impulsivity and inconsistency and generally have uneven patterns of intellectual functioning and difficulties using their skills in other instances, areas, or places. They often have exceptional skills in one or more areas such as memory, math, music, or repetitive mechanical abilities.

Autism is an umbrella term for a number of unusual and persistent characteristics, some of which appear in some individuals, some of which do not. There is no definitive test for autism, only some common characteristics by which to make a diagnosis.

Scientists now believe that they have uncovered a genetic link to some mentally debilitating disorders. A genetic defect called Fragile X Syndrome is believed to be responsible for some instances of "mental retardation" in families, and it has been suggested that some cases of autism are a result of Fragile X Syndrome. The reported occurrence of this gene is extremely rare, but it appears that the incidence of autism is suddenly on the rise.

The incidence of attention deficit disorder (with or without hyperactivity) is also on the rise. This disorder, like autism, occurs five times more frequently in males than in females. It is also distributed among all races, nationalities, and social classes. Its causes are unknown. There has been speculation that genetic factors, viruses, imbalances of certain chemicals in the brain, and environmental factors may be involved.

There is research that shows that children with these unusual handicaps typically do not do well in later years. They drop out of school more frequently. They have extremely low self-esteem.

They tend to abuse alcohol and drugs. They tend to be more physically aggressive and are much less likely to be skilled in any one area. They commit suicide more frequently. They commit crimes more frequently. And they often end up being supported by social programs (*i.e.*, social assistance, handicap pensions, welfare, job training programs, unemployment programs, detention centres, and penitentiaries). They are probably many of the homeless — victims of subtle and not-so-subtle mental handicaps.

We know little about the cause of psychological and mental problems such as conduct disorder, antisocial behavior, minimal brain dysfunction, attention deficit and hyperactivity disorder, pervasive developmental disorder, and autism. They appear to have multifactorial etiologies — that means there are several different causes that can give you the same symptoms. And the particular symptoms present in any case reflect the part of the brain that has been injured or damaged rather than the specific cause of injury.

With this in mind, we can see where a child may suffer from a debilitating illness such as encephalitis at an early age, and may end up with minimal brain dysfunction, conduct disorder, or pervasive developmental disorder. In fact, by definition, pervasive development disorder is a collection of syndromes that appear after the age of three where there has been a history of normal development up until that point. Frequently some kind of illness, trauma, or a marked change in behavior suggestive of a dramatic change has occurred in these children. Typically the comment is made, "Johnny was developing normally until such and such an age and then we noticed that his behavior changed. He became different. He became irritable, resisted contact, and was not as responsive as he was prior to that. His interaction with other children changed as well."

What is more confusing is when the changes have been more gradual and the parent reflects by saying, "Yes, he seemed to be normal when I look back to the first year or two but it wasn't until he was four years old that I noticed that he just wasn't learning things as quickly as some of his friends."

Children are sent to various social workers, psychologists, and psychiatrists who have developed batteries of tests which assess levels of physical, behavioral, cognitive, and emotional development and on the basis of these tests, children are categorized with labels such as attention deficit disorder, hyperactivity disorder or social adjustment disorder. They are then entered into therapeutic programs which rely upon the use of drugs such as Ritalin or a combination of drugs and behavioral modification.

It is reasonable to assume that children who are intellectually impaired will at some point develop behavioral disorders that will need to be addressed. In cases of severe intellectual impairment, the family will need to be counselled and supported. What we can't agree with is the ominous fact that up to 10 percent of our children need to be medicated with Ritalin and Ritalin-like stimulants.

There are now children in every school classroom, often many in each classroom, who are medicated with amphetamines and/or anti-depressants every day of their lives until adulthood so that they can sit in a classroom and be participants instead of distractions to the normal routine. Children as young as three years old need to be prescribed these potentially harmful medications. What do we know about these drugs?

First of all, Ritalin (methylphenidate) is a stimulant similar to "speed." It is commonly prescribed for attention deficit hyperactivity disorder, minimal brain dysfunction, hyperkinetic child syndrome, minimal brain damage, minimal cerebral dysfunction, and minor cerebral dysfunction. These disorders are characterized by symptoms such as distractibility, short attention span, hyperactivity, emotional instability, and impulsivity. Children with these disorders have difficulty with social adjustment and academic performance. When one looks upon this plethora of indications, and the lack of knowledge we have about these conditions at the purely scientific level, it is no wonder that this drug is a natural for abuse.

Often it seems to be the only thing that works. It seems a Godsend. Yet in some cases it exacerbates or exaggerates symptoms of behavior and thought disturbance. Hyperactivity can in fact be made worse. It can produce seizures by lowering the seizure threshold. It can lead to an increase in drug tolerance and psycho-logical dependence, otherwise known as addiction. It can result in frank psychotic decompensation with hallucinations and delu-sions. It can cause severe depression, insomnia, loss of weight, cardiac symptoms of angina and rhythm disturbances, hair loss, suppressed production of blood cells, and allergic reactions. There are other side effects associated with these medications but per-haps a logical way to think about them is to realize that they are metabolic stimulants and, as such, they accelerate the process of free radical damage and can result in signs of accelerated aging, particularly of the circulatory system. Accelerated hardening of the arteries and hypertension have been identified in earlier research with amphetamine-like medications.

So why is nobody asking, "If 10 percent of our children are receiving this type of medication, what is going on? What is the underlying factor that is causing this? Why have we not been able to identify the cause?"

These disorders have similar characteristics to those of chronic metal toxicity. We have to wonder if sometimes physicians are too concerned about looking for more exotic causes like genetic mutations for these neurological problems, when pollution and other environmental factors could be at work.

Medical literature has already established a positive correlation between high lead or cadmium burden in children and the pres-ence of learning disabilities and hyperactivity. There is also infor-mation available that tells us in no uncertain terms that pollutants such as lead, mercury, cadmium, insecticides, and herbicides are known to be a causative factor in many cases of attention deficit disorder and hyperactivity. This is not at all new. So why is no one testing for heavy metals in children that display these disorders? And when the incidence is rising so steadily and affecting the intelligence and mentality of these affected children, why aren't we looking at better, more effective methods of evaluating their body burden of metals?

Glossary

Acute — When used in this book in reference to toxicity, this means a rapid, severe, intense onset of symptoms due to recent excessive exposure to metals.

Affinity — An attraction between two substances, or the force which causes a substance to join with one particular substance rather than another.

Alloy — A metallic compound, a mixture of two or more metals.

Aluminum (Al) — A very light-weight, malleable metal of silvery white colour.

Alzheimer's disease — A progressive form of dementia occurring in middle age or later, for which there is no known cure. The cause is unknown. It is associated with diffuse or widespread degeneration of the brain.

Amygdala — An almond-shaped mass of grey matter, deep inside the brain, which is responsible for functions concerned with mood, feeling, instinct, and recent memory.

Anafranil (clomipramine HCL) — An antidepressant that has been found useful in the treatment of primary depressive illness. Its mild sedative effect may be helpful in alleviating anxiety.

Anemia — A deficiency in the blood, either in quality or quantity, usually involving red blood cells or hemoglobin.

Angina — Spasmodic, choking, or suffocating pain, now used almost exclusively to refer to a pain in the heart muscle.

Antibody — A protein produced in the body in response to a foreign agent (antigen) which reacts to overcome the toxic effects of the antigen.

Antigen — Any substance not normally present in the body which stimulates production of an antibody.

Arsenic (As) — A medicinal and poisonous metal which is brittle and greyish with a garlicky odor.

Atherosclerosis — A disease of the arteries in which fatty plaques develop on their inner walls with eventual obstruction of blood flow. Also called hardening of the arteries.

Attention deficit disorder (ADD or ADHD) — A developmental disorder.

The ADD label is applied when eight or more of the following symptoms are noticeable for more than six months: a child is restless, has difficulty remaining seated when required to do so, is easily distracted, has difficulty awaiting turns, blurts out answers to questions before they are completed, has difficulty following instructions, can not sustain attention in tasks or at play, shifts frequently from one activity to another, has difficulty playing quietly, talks excessively, frequently interrupts or intrudes, seems not to listen to what is being said, often loses things, engages in physically dangerous activities without considering consequences. ADD children are distinguished from others by the number of behaviors present, the length of time they continue, and the degree to which they are evident. See Appendix for more information.

Autism — A rare, life-long developmental disability that is believed to be present at birth in which a person is dominated by self-centered trends of thought or behavior which are not affected by external information. See Appendix for more information.

Auto-immune response — An immune response in which a person's cells or antibodies react to and attack his or her own body.

Behavioral modification — A program to change a person's conduct or activity, usually used for behavioral problems or inappropriate activity.

Biopsy — The removal of tissue from a living body for the purpose of examination and diagnosis.

Blood-brain barrier — A semipermeable membrane which keeps the circulating blood separate from the tissue surrounding the brain cells. It allows necessary nutrients in solution to pass through but excludes larger molecules.

Blood lead level — The amount of lead that is in a person's blood at any given time.

Body burden — In this book, body burden refers specifically to the quantity of lead and other metals that has accumulated in a person's body tissues, as opposed to the amount present in the blood.

British Anti-Lewisite (BAL) — A chelating agent specifically made as an antidote to arsenic-based Lewisite — a poison gas used as a weapon in war.

Cadmium (Cd) — A poisonous, silvery metal resembling tin.

Calcium (Ca) — A silvery yellow mineral important in the process of blood clotting.

Cardiovascular system — The body system made up of the heart and blood vessels (arteries and veins).

Catalyst — A substance that initiates a chemical reaction but is itself unchanged at the end of the chemical reaction. The catalysts in biochemical reactions are enzymes.

Causative factor — An agent or element that is responsible for the production of a result, as, for example, aluminum could be a causative factor for childhood hyperactivity.

Central nervous system — The control center of the nervous system, composed of the brain and spinal cord, which receives input from the peripheral nervous system.

Cerebellum — The largest part of the hindbrain which is responsible for maintaining muscle tone, balance, and voluntary muscle control.

Cerebral cortex — The intricately folded outer layer of the cerebrum which makes up 40 percent of the brain by weight and is responsible for consciousness, perception, memory, thought, mental ability, intellect, and voluntary activity.

Chelating agent / chelator — A chemical compound that forms complexes by binding to metal ions. When used for medical purposes, metals present in the body are bound to the drug and excreted safely from the body.

Chelation — The process of removing metal ions from body tissues by binding them with a synthetic compound which can be safely excreted from the body.

Chromium (Cr) — A blue-whitish, brittle metal.

Chronic — When used in this book in reference to toxicity, this means a slow, gradual onset of symptoms due to long-term, low-level exposure to metals.

Clonidine — A medication used for extreme behavioral problems and agitation.

Cobalt (Co) — A silvery white metal.

Co-factors — An element or substance with which another must unite in order to function. For example, trace minerals and vitamins are co-factors with enzymes in chemical reactions.

Cognitive function — The ability to gain knowledge from personal experience, or the ability to reason and learn from perceiving, thinking, and experiencing.

Colic — Acute abdominal pain.

Coordination chemistry — A branch of chemistry that studies the complexing of positively charged atoms within molecules based on the sharing of electrons.

Copper (Cu) — A reddish malleable metal.

Cuprimine (penicillamine) — A chelating agent used largely for removal of copper from the body (*e.g.*, Wilson's disease) and also for rheumatoid arthritis and chronic lead poisoning.

Decilitre (dl) — One tenth of a litre.

Demineralization — The process where the body pulls minerals out of the bones to maintain a proper balance in the blood (*e.g.*, during pregnancy).

Demyelination — A disease process which selectively damages the myelin sheaths that protect nerves of the central or peripheral nervous system.

Desferal (desferoxamine) — An oral chelating agent.

Detoxification — Removing toxins or poisons from the body.

Developmental delay — A delay or ceasing of mental, physical, and social growth at some stage before such growth is normally completed.

DMPS (dimercaptopropanesulfonic acid) — An oral chelating agent.

DMSA (dimercaptosuccinic acid) — An oral chelating agent.

DNA (deoxyribonucleic acid) — The basic substance of genes which carry the genetic code controlling development of an organism.

Double-blind studies — A comparison of the outcome between two or more groups of patients that are deliberately subjected to different regimens — one being a "control group" with no active treatment, the other group receiving treatment.

DSM-III-R (Diagnostic and Statistical Manual of Mental Disorders) — A guide produced by the American Psychiatric Association used by physicians, psychologists, psychiatrists etc. to diagnose mental handicaps and illnesses.

Dysfunctional — Disturbed, impaired, or abnormal functioning of an organ or organism.

Dyslexia — An inability to comprehend written language.

EDTA (ethylene diamine tetracetic acid) — A compound used as a chelating agent in the treatment of several different metals.

Elemental hair analysis — Analysis of hair by atomic absorption spectography which measures the quantities of elements present.

Encephalopathy — Any of various diseases that affect the functioning of the brain.

Enzymes — Proteins that promote biochemical reactions in living organisms.

Epidemiology — The study of the occurence of factors which influence the frequency and distribution of specific diseases.

Etiological factor — The cause of a specific disease.

Fragile X Syndrome — A genetic mutation believed to be responsible for profound mental retardation in families.

Fraternal twins — Twins who do not necessarily resemble each other as they develop from two fertilized eggs rather than one.

Free radical — A molecule with an unpaired electron in its outer atomic orbit which is highly unstable and will react with any substance in its path (responsible for damaging cells by this process in the body). These reactions rapidly create new unbalanced atoms, thereby magnifying the potential for damage in body cells/structures.

Gastro-intestinal system — The body system made up of the stomach and intestines.

Gout — A disease in which uric acid appears in excessive quantities in the blood and may be deposited in the joints and other tissues causing swelling, inflammation, and pain in the joints.

Half-life — The time in which one-half the quantity of an element is eliminated by excretion or absorption from, for example, the blood or body tissues.

Hematemesis — The vomiting of blood.

Hemochromatosis — A disorder of iron metabolism where excess iron is deposited in tissues causing changes in skin pigment, cirrhosis of the liver, and decreased carbohydrate tolerance. Often referred to as "iron storage disease."

Hemoglobin — The molecule that transports oxygen through the bloodstream to organs and tissues.

Hippocampus — A portion of the floor of the lateral ventricle of the brain which contains complex foldings of cortical tissue. This is one of the brain's most primitve parts and controls physical behavior governed by emotions and instinct.

Hyperactivity — Abnormally increased activity which can result from brain damage or psychosis. In children, hyperactivity is characterized by constant motion and, usually, distractibility and low frustration thresholds.

Hypertension — Excessive pressure of the blood against arterial walls, otherwise known as high blood pressure.

Immune system — The body's system which protects against the invasion of foreign bodies (antigens).

Immunosuppression — A process which inhibits the formation of antibodies to combat antigens that may be present in the body.

Insult — A trauma or injury which causes damage to body organs or mental development.

Integrity — The state of being whole, entire, or unimpaired.

Intravenous — Pertaining to the vein, this also refers to the process of giving medication to a patient through an injection into a vein.

Ion — An atom that has a net positive or negative charge due to a loss or gain of electrons.

Iron (Fe) — A metal essential to life as it is a vital component in the transfer of oxygen in the body.

Keratinous structure — The principal constituent of skin, hair, nails, and the enamel of the teeth.

Leaching — The process by which water can dissolve and remove substances (like metals) from soil or pipes through which it passes.

Lead (Pb) — A soft, heavy, bluish-grey metal that forms several poisonous compounds.

Lithium (Li) — An essential metal required in humans for normal mental processes.

Macrophages — Cells that remove foreign debris from body tissues.

Malleability — The property of a substance which allows it to withstand hammering, pressing, or rolling into thin sheets without breaking.

Manganese (Mn) — A metal resembling iron which is essential for some enzyme functions in the body.

Mercury (Hg) — A poisonous, heavy, silvery metal that is liquid at room temperature.

Metabolism — The physical and chemical processes in an organism by which cells are produced, maintained, and destroyed, and by which energy is made available for the body's functioning. The food we eat and the air we breathe are necessary for metabolic processes.

Metal — Any of a group of elements characterized by their luster, malleability, ductility, and conductivity of electricity and heat.

Metallothionein — A protein which is secreted by the placenta and can bind with cadmium and some other heavy metals to block their transport to the fetus.

Microgram (μg) — One one-millionth of a gram.

Mineral — An inorganic substance usually present in Earth's crust. The difference between trace elements and minerals is that minerals actually form a part of a body structure whereas trace elements play an important role in enzyme reactions but do not form body structures.

Mole — The molecular weight of a substance expressed in grams.

Molybdenum (Mo) — A hard, silvery white metal.

Morphology — The branch of biology dealing with the form and structure of living organisms.

Motor nerve — A nerve that affects or produces movement.

Motor skill — The ability to move and to control the movement of the body. Fine motor skills refers to the ability, for example, to use scissors or do other exacting activities with the hands.

Multiple sclerosis — A chronic disease of the nervous system affecting young and middle-aged adults. Myelin sheaths surrounding nerves in the brain and spinal cord become damaged, which affects functioning of the nerves involved. Symptoms include unsteady gait, shaky movements of limbs, rapid involuntary movements of eyes, defects in speech pronunciation, and spastic weakness. The underlying cause is unknown.

Mutagenic — Something that can cause an increased rate of mutation when applied to cells or organisms. For example, something that will affect the DNA of a cell.

Neurological disorder — A malfunction of the nervous system where messages from the brain are not transmitted properly to various parts of the body.

Neurology — The branch of medical science which deals with the nervous system.

Neurotoxin — A substance that is destructive of or poisonous to nerve tissue.

New growth hair sample — Hair removed from close to the scalp, generally the first inch of growth from the scalp, to be used for elemental analysis.

Nickel (Ni) — A silver-white metal.

Osteoporosis — A bone disease which leads to inadequate calcium absorption into bone and results in thinning of the skeleton.

Oxidation — To combine or cause to combine with oxygen. The chemical reaction where electrons are removed from atoms of the substance being oxidized.

Parkinson's disease — A disorder of middle-aged and elderly people characterized by tremor, rigidity, slowness of movements and speech, and a masklike, expressionless face. It affects the basal ganglia of the brain but the underlying cause is unknown.

Penicillamine (Cuprimine) — A chelating agent commonly used in the treatment of Wilson's disease, also for lead poisoning and rheumatoid arthritis.

Peripheral nervous system — A system of nerves that connects outer parts of the body to the central nervous system.

Pervasive development disorder — A collection of developmental syndromes that seems to occur after age three when there has been a history of normal development up to that point.

pH — A measurement of the concentration of hydrogen ions in a solution. A pH of 7 is neutral. Solutions with a pH of less than 7 are acidic; greater than 7 are alkaline.

Phosphorous (P) — A nonmetallic, poisonous, inflammable element.

Photophobia — An abnormal dread or intolerance of light.

Physiology — The science which studies the functioning of living organisms and their component parts, and the physical and chemical factors involved.

Pica — The licking, chewing, or eating of non-food substances such as dirt, painted wood surfaces and objects, toys, etc.

Protein — Any of a group of complex organic nitrogen-containing compounds that are required for all life processes.

Provocative urine sample — A urine sample obtained after the administration of a chelating agent.

Psychotic — Pertaining to a mental disorder characterized by loss of contact with reality and derangement of personality, often accompanied by delusions, hallucinations, or illusions.

Reactive oxygen toxic species (ROTS) — Free radicals. Highly unstable and reactive molecules.

Ritalin (methylphenidate HCL) — A central nervous system stimulant whose mode of action is not completely understood. Presumably it activates the brain stem arousal system and cortex to produce a stimulant effect.

Sequester — To lodge in body tissue. For example, lead atoms lodged in human bones are said to be sequestered.

Silicon (Si) — A nonmetallic light element.

Silver (Ag) — A white, soft, malleable metal.

Soft tissues — The collective name for body tissues including muscular, connective, vascular, fatty, and fibrous tissues as opposed to the bones.

Stimulation — The act or process of exciting the brain or sense organs to action. Self-stimulation involves exciting the brain as an end in itself.

Strontium (Sr) — A dark yellowish metal.

Synapses — The junction between two adjacent nerve cells, where a nervous impulse is transmitted from one nerve cell to another.

Syndrome — A set of symptoms which occur together.

Synergistic effect — The combined action of two substances that, when interacting with each other, produce increased effect which is greater than the sum of the effects of the substances when acting separately.

Teratogenic — An agent or factor that causes physical abnormalities in a developing fetus.

Tin (Sn) — A white malleable metal.

Toxicity — The quality of being poisonous or the degree to which a substance is poisonous.

Trace elements — Elements found in plants and animals in minuscule quantities that are believed to be critical factors in enzyme reactions.

Uric acid — A component of urine that is the end product of nucleic acid metabolism or oxidation. Uric acid crystals deposited in joints cause gout.

Vanadium (V) — A rare, grey metal.

Wilson's disease — A genetically acquired disease that results in the excessive accumulation of copper in various tissues, particularly the kidney, liver, brain, and red blood cells. Also known as "copper storage disease."

X-ray fluorescence — A testing method which uses x-rays to provide a relatively accurate measure of lead (and potentially other metal) content in bone.

Zinc (Zn) — A blue-white metal.

Bibliography

A long-term burden — Higher lead, lower intelligence. *Consumer Reports* 58, no. 2 (1993).

A summary of pharmocological and clinical data: Chemet-Succimer. Pamphlet from McNeil Consumer Products Co., 1991.

Aaseth, J., J. Alexander, and N. Rakerud. Treatment of mercuric chloride poisoning with dimercaptosuccinic acid and diuretics: Preliminary studies. *Journal of Toxicology* 19, no. 2 (1982).

Allison, M. Lead poisoning — Not just for kids. *Harvard Health Letter* 17, no. 7 (1992).

Altman, R. *The complete book of home environmental hazards — And how to get rid of them.* New York, NY: Facts on File, 1990.

American Academy of Pediatrics advises lead screening for children. *FDA Consumer* 27, no. 6 (1993).

American Psychiatric Association. *Diagnostic and statistical manual of mental disorders* 3d ed., rev. Washington, DC: American Psychiatric Association, 1987.

Baghurst, P.A., A. McMichael, N.R. Wigg, G.V. Vimpani, E.F. Robertson, R.J. Roberts, S.L. Tong. Environmental exposure to lead and children's intelligence at the age of seven years. *New England Journal of Medicine* 327, no. 18 (1992).

Blaurock-Busch, E. Mineral imbalances in pregnant mothers and their newborn. *Journal of Orthomolecular Medicine* 5, no. 3 (1990).

Bradford, R.W., H.W. Allen, and M.L. Culbert. *Oxidology — The study of reactive oxygen toxic species (ROTS) and their metabolism in health and disease.* Los Altos, CA: Robert W. Bradford Foundation, 1985.

Campbell, J.D. Hair analysis: A diagnostic tool for measuring mineral status in humans. *Journal of Orthomolecular Psychiatry* 14, no. 4 (1985).

Castleman, M. Lead again. *Sierra* 77 (July/August 1992).

Centers for Disease Control. *Preventing lead poisoning in young children: A statement by the Centers for Disease Control.* CDC report no. 99-2230 (1991).

Children in peril. *Newsweek* 117, no. 26 (1991).

Coffel, S. *But not a drop to drink! The lifesaving guide to good water.* New York, NY: Ballantine Books, 1989.

Cranton, E.M. Interpretation of trace and toxic element levels in human hair. *Journal of Advancement in Medicine* 2, no. 1/2 (1989).

Cranton, E.M., and J.P. Frackelton. Free-radical pathology in age-associated diseases: Treatment with EDTA chelation, nutrition, and antioxidants. *Journal of Holistic Medicine* 6, no. 1 (1984).

Cranton, E.M., Z.X. Liu, and I.M. Smith. Urinary trace and toxic elements and minerals in untimed urine specimens relative to urine creatinine, part II: Evoked increase in excretion following intravenous EDTA. *Journal of Advancement in Medicine* 2, no. 1/2 (1989).

Cromwell, P.E., B.R. Abadie, J.T. Stephens, and M. Kyler. Hair mineral analysis: Biochemical imbalances and violent criminal behavior. *Psychological Reports* 64, no. 1 (1989).

Daunderer, M. Improvement of nerve and immunological damages. *American Journal of Prebiotic Dentistry and Medicine* (January/March 1991).

Foster, H.D. Aluminum and health. *Journal of Orthomolecular Medicine* 7, no. 4 (1992).

Gottschalk, L.A., T. Rebello, M.S. Buchbaum, H.G. Tucker, and E.L. Hodges. Abnormalities in hair trace elements as indicators of aberrant behavior. *Comprehensive Psychiatry* 32, no. 3 (1991).

Greater Vancouver Regional District. Drinking water quality improvements. *Reflections* 1, no. 1 (1992).

Green, R.G. Hyperactivity and the learning disabled child. *Journal of Orthomolecular Psychiatry* 9, no. 2 (1980).

―――. Diagnosis and treatment of perceptual dysfunctions, hyperactivity, and learning disabilities. *Journal of Orthomolecular Psychiatry* 10, no. 3 (1981).

Halstead, B.W. *The scientific basis of EDTA chelation therapy.* Colton, CA: Golden Quill Publishers, 1979.

Hammer, D.I., J.F. Finklea, R.H. Hendricks, T.A. Hinners, W.B. Riggan, and C.M. Shy. Trace metals in human hair as a simple epidemiological monitor of environmental exposure. In *Trace Substances in Environmental Health,* D.D. Hemphill, ed. Columbia, MO: University of Missouri, 1972.

Hoffer, A. Children with learning and behavioral disorders. *Journal of Orthomolecular Medicine* 5, no. 3 (1976).

Hotz, M.C.B., ed. *Health effects of lead.* Ottawa, ON: Royal Society of Canada Commisssion on Lead in the Environment, 1986.

How to avoid exposure to lead. *C.Q. Researcher* 2, no. 23 (1992).

Is there lead in your water? *Consumer Reports* 58, no. 2 (1993).

Iyengar, G.V., W.E. Kollmer, and H.J.M. Bowen. *The elemental composition of human tissues and body fluids: A compilation of values for adults.* New York, NY: Verlag Chemie, 1978.

Jenkins, D.W. *Biological monitoring of toxic trace metals.* Environmental Protection Agency report no. 600/3-80-089 (1980).

Kopito, L., A.M. Dilley, II. Shwachman. Chronic plumbism in children. *Journal of the American Medical Association* 209, no. 2 (1969).

Kopito, L., R.K. Byers, H. Shwachman. Lead in hair of children with chronic lead poisoning. *New England Journal of Medicine* 276, no. 17 (1967).

LaDou, J., ed. *Occupational medicine.* Norwalk CT: Appleton and Lange, 1990.

Lead. *Science and technology* 6. New York, NY: McGraw-Hill, 1982.

Lead-heads. *The Economist* 321, no. 7730 (1991).

Lead poisoning — Are children suffering because of weak prevention efforts? *C.Q. Researcher* 2 (June 19, 1992).

Lead poisoning reversible. *Arizona Republic* (April 7, 1993).

Levine, S.A., and P.M. Kidd. *Antioxidant adaptation: Its role in free radical pathology.* San Leandro, CA: Biocurrents Division, Allergy Research Group, 1985.

Marlowe, M. Low level aluminum exposure and childhood motor performance. *Journal of Orthomolecular Medicine* 7, no. 3 (1992).

Marlowe, M., C. Moon, J. Errera, and J. Stellern. Hair mineral content as a predictor of mental retardation. *Journal of Orthomolecular Psychiatry* 12, no. 1 (1983).

Marlowe, M., C. Moon, J. Errera, J. Jacobs, M. Brunson, J. Stellern, C. Schroeder. Low mercury levels and childhood intelligence. *Journal of Orthomolecular Medicine* 1, no. 1 (1986).

Marlowe, M., J. Errera, and J.C. Case. Hair selenium levels and children's classroom behavior. *Journal of Orthomolecular Medicine* 1, no. 2 (1986).

Marlowe, M., J. Errera, J. Jacobs. Increased lead and cadmium burdens among mentally retarded children and children with borderline intelligence. *American Journal of Mental Deficiency* 87, no. 5 (1983).

Marlowe, M., J. Errera, J. Stellern, and D. Beck. Lead and mercury levels in emotionally disturbed children. *Journal of Orthomolecular Psychiatry* 12, no. 4 (1983).

Minder, B., E.A. Das-Smaal, E. Brand, and J.F. Orlebeke. Exposure to lead and specific attentional problems in schoolchildren. *Journal of Learning Disabilities* 27, no. 6 (1994).

Moon, C., M. Marlowe, and J. Errera. Main and interaction effects of metallic pollutants on cognitive functioning. *Journal of Learning Disabilities* 18, no. 4 (1985).

Needleman, H.L., and P.J. Landrigan. *Raising children toxic free: How to keep your child safe from lead, asbestos, pesticides, and other environmental hazards.* New York, NY: Farrar, Straus and Giroux, 1994.

Needleman, H.L., C. Gunnoe, A. Leviton, R. Reed, H. Peresie, C. Maher, and P. Barrett. Deficits in psychologic and classroom performance of children with elevated dentine lead levels. *New England Journal of Medicine* 300, no. 13 (1979).

Oliver, B. The children who should have been passing but didn't. *Journal of Orthomolecular Psychiatry* 12, no. 3 (1983).

Pangborn, J.B. *Mechanisms of detoxification and procedures for detoxification.* Chicago, IL: Doctor's Data Inc. and Bionostics Inc., 1994.

Pear, R. U.S. orders testing of poor children for lead poisoning. *New York Times* (September 13, 1992).

Pihl, R.O., and M. Parkes. Hair element content in learning disabled children. *Science* 198, no. 4313 (1977).

Piomelli, S., J.F. Rosen, J. Chisholm Jr., and J.W. Graef. Management of childhood lead poisoning. *Journal of Pediatrics* 1988.

Pleva, J. Mercury poisoning from dental amalgam. *Journal of Orthomolecular Psychiatry* 12, no. 3 (1983).

Pueschel, S. Neurological and psychomotor functions in children with an increased lead burden. *Environmental Health Perspectives* 1, no. 7 (1974).

Pueschel, S.M., L. Kopito, and H. Schwachman. Children with an increased lead burden — A screening and follow-up study. *Journal of the American Medical Association* 222, no. 4 (1972).

Rees, E.L. Aluminum toxicity as indicated by hair analysis. *Journal of Orthomolecular Psychiatry* 8, no. 1 (1979).

Rice, D.C. Behavioral deficit (delayed matching to sample) in monkeys exposed from birth to low levels of lead. *Toxicology and Applied Pharmacology* 75, no. 2 (1984).

————. Chronic low-lead exposure from birth produces deficits in discrimination reversal in monkeys. *Toxicology and Applied Pharmacology* 77, no. 2 (1985).

Rice, D.C., and S.G. Gilbert. Low-lead exposure from birth produces behavioral toxicity (DRL) in monkeys. *Toxicology and Applied Pharmacology* 80, no. 3 (1985).

Rice, D.C., S.G. Gilbert, and R.F. Willes. Neonatal low-level lead exposure in monkeys: locomotor activity, schedule-controlled behaviors and the effects of amphetamine. *Toxicology and Applied Pharmacology* 51, no. 3 (1979).

Rice, D.C. and R.F. Willes. Neonatal low-lead exposure in monkeys (*Macaca fascicularis*): Effect on two-choice non-spatial form discrimination. *Journal of Environmental Pathology and Toxicology* 2 (1979).

Rimland, B., and G.E. Larson. Hair mineral analysis and behavior: An analysis of 51 studies. *Journal of Learning Disabilities* 16, no. 5 (1983).

Ruff, A.H., and P.E. Bijur. The effects of low to moderate lead levels on neurobehavioral functioning in children: Toward a conceptual model. *Developmental And Behavioral Pediatrics* 10, no. 2 (1989).

Ruff, A.H., P.E. Bijur, M. Markowitz, Y.C. Ma, and J.F. Rosen. Declining blood lead levels and cognitive changes in moderately lead-poisoned children. *Journal of the American Medical Association* 269, no. 13 (1993).

Schauss, A.G., and C.E. Simonsen. A critical analysis of the diets of chronic juvenile offenders, part 1. *Journal of Orthomolecular Psychiatry* 8, no. 3 (1979).

Schrauzer, G.N., and K.P. Shrestha. Lithium in drinking water and the incidences of crimes, suicides, and arrests related to drug addictions. *Biological Trace Element Research* 25, no. 2 (1990).

Schubert, J., E.J. Riley, and S.A. Tyler. Combined effects in toxicology — A rapid systematic testing procedure: cadmium, mercury, and lead. *Journal of Toxicology and Environmental Health* 4, no. 5/6 (1978).

Setterberg, F., and L. Shavelson. *Toxic Nation.* New York, NY: Wiley and Sons, Inc., 1993.

Smith, B.L. Cardiovascular risk as related to an element pattern in hair. *Trace Elements in Medicine* 4, no. 3 (1987).

Smith, B. Organic foods vs supermarket foods: Element levels. *Journal of Applied Nutrition* 45, no. 1 (1993).

Thatcher, R.W., et al. Evoked potentials related to hair cadmium and lead in children. *New York Academy of Science* 425 (1984).

The news on lead. *Berkeley Wellness Letter* (November 1993).

Trace metals in hair are easier to study. *Journal of the American Medical Association* 215, no. 3 (1971).

U.S. Department of Health and Human Services. *Strategic plan for the elimination of childhood lead poisoning.* Atlanta, GA: Centers for Disease Control, 1991.

U.S. Department of Housing and Urban Development. *Comprehensive and workable plan for the abatement of lead-based paint in privately owned housing: Report to Congress.* Washington, DC: HUD, 1990.

U.S. Environmental Protection Agency. Toxic trace metals in mammalian hair and nails. EPA report no. 600/4-79-049 (1979).

———. *Strategy for reducing lead exposures: Report to Congress.* (1991).

———. *Lead Poisoning and Your Child.* EPA report no. 800-B-92-0002 (1992).

Wallace, B., and K. Cooper. *The citizen's guide to lead.* Toronto, ON: NC Press, 1986.

Watts, D.L. The nutritional relationships of chromium. *Journal of Orthomolecular Medicine* 4, no. 1 (1989).

———. The nutritional relationships of copper. *Journal of Orthomolecular Medicine* 4, no. 2 (1989).

Why lead may leave kids short. *Science News* 142, no. 9 (1992).

Wisner, R.M., D. Root, M. Shields, and S.L. Beckmann. Neurotoxicity and toxic body burdens: Relationship and treatment potentials. In *Proceedings of the International Conference on Peripheral Nerve Toxicity,* 1993.

Index

absorption: children *vs.* adults 62
acetyl choline 138
acetyl choline transferase 138
acid rain 120, 121, 147, 160
acid water 89, 120, 121, 130, 147, 160
acidic food 163, 166
acute lead toxicity: blood tests 78; guidelines (table) 79
acute metal toxicity: symptoms 64, 78
adrenalin 138
air pollution 90, 121, 122, 128, 147, 160; lead 119
allergies 76
Alliance to End Childhood Lead Poisoning 53, 150
aluminum 126, 137, 146, 166; and brain 77; and vision 115; sources 139
Alzheimer's disease 138
American College for Advancement in Medicine 112, 113
American Psychiatric Association 51
ammonia 139
amino acids 76
Anafranil 15, 22
anemia 41, 58, 64, 74, 79, 102, 108, 128, 138, 141, 143, 144
antimony 125
arsene 137
arsenic 90, 125, 136, 146, 149; and hair analysis 69; and lead 136; production 137; sources 137
asthma 128

atherosclerosis 58, 136, 141, 142; and chelation 170; and EDTA 76
attention deficit disorder 15, 80, 83, 98, 104; causes 37; diagnosis 187; occurrence 192; suggested causes 192; testing 36
autism 15, 51, 80, 104; causes 37, 191; costs 181; description 191; occurrence 18, 191; responds to metal detoxification 169; testing 36
autistic tendencies 65, 83, 98, 191; diagnosis of 187
automobile emissions 89, 90, 93, 105, 109, 114, 121, 122, 130, 156, 164, 176

Baghurst, Peter A. 54
barium 125
batteries 119, 124, 135, 137, 145, 160, 165; nicad 130
behavior disorders 43, 47, 49, 53, 58, 64, 65, 83, 133, 145; and chronic toxicity 64; and lead 53; misdiagnosis 66
behavior modification 22, 30
Bersworth, Frederick 75
beryllium 125
beta dopamine hydroxylase 138
Bijur, Polly 49, 100
birth defects 128
blood lead: acute *vs.* chronic toxicity 57, 172, 175; and body burden 48, 80; changes in acceptable levels 44, 67, 78, 174; in umbilical cord 63; missing

Metal Detox Medical Services offers

1 Hair elemental analysis sample kit and instructions. Testing for 21 elements will be performed by a certified laboratory for about US$25. Results will be returned within 3 to 4 weeks by Metal Detox (lab will not return results directly to client). Although hair elemental analysis is not to be used alone as a diagnostic tool, it can help to reveal the need for more indepth investigation.

___ Hair analysis kit(s) CDN$10 (Outside Canada US$8)

2. Additional copies of *Turning Lead Into Gold*. (Special rates for orders of 10 or more copies available on request.)

___ Copy(ies) of *Turning Lead Into Gold* @ CDN$22 (In U.S. US$20; overseas US$21)

Prices cover materials, postage, handling, and taxes. Allow 3 weeks for delivery. Please make cheques or money orders payable to:

Metal Detox Medical Services Inc., PO Box 16096, 3017 Mountain Highway, North Vancouver, B. C. V7K 3A5 Canada

Name _____

Name on sample _____

Address _____

_____

Province/State _____ Code _____ Country _____

3. Detailed guidelines for patients, physicians, and healthcare providers regarding protocols for diagnosis and treatment of heavy metal toxicities using chelating agents are available for US$20. Price covers cost of materials, postage, handling, and taxes. Please allow 3 weeks for delivery. Make cheques or money orders in US funds payable to:

Metal Detox Medical Services Inc., 1733 H Street, Suite 330-157, Blaine, Washington USA 98230-5107

Please send ___ Guideline Manual(s) for diagnosis and treatment of heavy metal toxicity to:

Name _____

Address _____

_____

Province/State _____ Code _____ Country _____